This book is due for return on or before the last date shown below.

ion
nes
ent
ing

Spires

drews

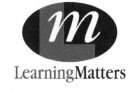

LearningMatters

First published in 2011 by Learning Matters Ltd

British Library Cataloguing in Publication Data
A CIP record for this book is available from the British Library

ISBN: 978 1 84445 845 5

This book is also available in the following ebook formats:

Adobe ebook: 978 1 84445 847 9
EPUB ebook: 978 1 84445 846 2
Kindle: 978 0 85725 047 6

Cover and text design by Toucan Design
Project Management by Diana Chambers
Typeset by Kelly Winter
Printed and bound in Great Britain by TJ International Ltd, Padstow, Cornwall

Learning Matters Ltd
20 Cathedral Yard
Exeter EX1 1HB
Tel: 01392 215560
E-mail: info@learningmatters.co.uk
www.learningmatters.co.uk

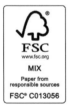

Contents

Foreword

The responsibility for the administration of medicines is one that is often viewed as a key function separating the registered nurse from other nursing roles. With science progressing at an ever-increasing rate in the field of pharmacology, the nurse's role in ensuring patients are treated with their prescribed medicines appropriately, accurately, safely and ethically is paramount.

This text will provide you with the foundation knowledge you require for your first year of the pre-registration nursing course. Beginning with an essential overview of mathematical principles, the authors will guide you safely through the maze of current medicines management in nursing practice. You will find plenty of practical examples to help you get to grips with the principles of pharmacokinetics and pharmacodynamics. Throughout the text are detailed and helpful explanations and, while the language of medicines and drugs may seem unfamiliar, the authors provide opportunities for you to practise using the terminology so that you will become confident and proficient.

You will have an opportunity to learn about alternative and complementary medicines, and broaden your understanding of treatment options for patients who are in pain. Because this text is by way of an overture on the subject, you will also be introduced to medicines management in specific field environments with relevant examples from adult, mental health, child health and learning disability fields. Further, separate, texts will follow in the series that will deal specifically and in detail on the requirements for these fields.

As with any subject in nursing, the needs of the patient remain uppermost. It could be possible when studying medicines management to get caught up in the fascination of pharmacology. However, the many activities and applied examples in this text firmly place the knowledge within a practical context and not as separate from the patient. The patient's condition and underlying health problems are never forgotten. That said, the way in which the authors tackle the subject make it seem fascinating and you will really be able to expand your nursing knowledge. Any curiosity you had about how medicines work will be well and truly satisfied after reading this excellent text.

Dr Shirley Bach
Series Editor

Introduction

Who is this book for?

This book is intended as an introductory book for first-year nursing students and is part of a mini-series that aims to equip students with the necessary knowledge and skills to become independent in medicines administration and drug calculation at the point of entry to the register. It will follow the Nursing and Midwifery Council Essential Skills Clusters and related proficiency standards with the aim of preparing students for medicines' assessments required to pass the first, and sometimes second, progression points in nursing degree programmes.

Although the book will assume a basic level of numeracy, it includes a chapter on mathematical skills and medicines dosage calculations for those who require revision or further practice. It introduces nursing students to the requirements for medicines management and patient education and sets this within the legal, professional and ethical framework to ensure safe and competent practice.

Book structure

The book has been designed to supplement your nursing studies and to be used for self-study. It is divided into seven easy-to-read chapters. The layout of the book enables you to dip in and out of chapters. It can be read through in a chapter order sequence or each chapter can be read as a stand-alone topic.

Chapter 1 provides an overview of the mathematical principles required to accurately and safely perform medicine dose calculations. It also looks at units of weight, volume and their equivalences.

Chapter 2 discusses legal, ethical and professional issues underpinning medicines management. Key legislation governing the supply, storage, dispensing and administration of medicines is explored. Ethical and professional considerations are discussed to enable you to understand how you should act when confronted with some tricky situations.

Chapter 3 describes the basic pharmacology of medicines and the factors impacting on their ability to work. It considers the route of administration and how this affects the pharmacodynamics and pharmacokinetics of medicines.

Chapter 4 looks at the role of medicines within holistic care. It discusses the use of a wide range of complementary and alternative methods to treat or manage a patient's illness, disease or health condition, including pain.

Chapter 5 focuses on the administration of medicines and the roles and responsibilities of the nurse in safe medicines management. It explores the use of documentation in recording and reporting processes. It also looks at issues that could compromise patient safety, such as anaphylaxis and polypharmacy, and those that can enhance concordance such as self-administration of medicines.

Chapter 6 explores a variety of issues and the pharmacological management of some medical conditions specific to each of the four fields of practice. It discusses the use of medical devices, the importance of getting the dose right for children, the management of pain in the patient who misuses opioids and gaining informed consent from patients with learning disabilities. Common medical conditions and their pharmacological management are also discussed.

Chapter 7 will help you understand how the interprofessional team contributes to medicines management.

Requirements for the NMC *Standards for Pre-registration Nursing Education* and the *Essential Skills Clusters*

The Nursing and Midwifery Council (NMC) has established standards of competence to be met by applicants to different parts of the register, and these are the standards it considers necessary for safe and effective practice. In addition to the competencies, the NMC has set out specific skills that nursing students must be able to perform at various points of an education programme. These are known as Essential Skills Clusters (ESCs). This book is structured so that it will help you to understand and meet the competencies and ESCs required for entry to the NMC register. The relevant competencies and ESCs are presented at the start of each chapter so that you can clearly see which ones the chapter addresses. There are *generic standards* that all nursing students, irrespective of their field, must achieve, and *field-specific standards* relating to each field of nursing: mental health, children's, learning disability and adult nursing. Most chapters have generic standards.

This book includes the latest standards, taken from *Standards for Pre-registration Nursing Education* (NMC, 2010a). For links to the pre-2010 standards, please visit the website for the book at **www.learningmatters.co.uk/nursing**.

Activities

Throughout the book you will find activities in the text that will help you to make sense of, and learn about, the material being presented by the authors.

Some activities ask you to reflect on aspects of practice, or your experience of it, or the people or situations you encounter. *Reflection* is an essential skill in nursing, and it helps you to understand the world around you and often to identify how things might be improved. Other activities will help you develop key skills, such as your ability to *think critically* about a topic in order to challenge received wisdom, or your ability to *research a topic and find appropriate information and evidence*, and to be able to *make decisions* using that evidence in situations that are often difficult and time-pressured. Finally, communication and working as part of a team are core to all nursing practice, and some activities will ask you to carry out activities or think about your *communication skills* to help develop these.

All the activities require you to take a break from reading the text, think through the issues presented and carry out some independent study, possibly using the internet. Where appropriate, there are sample answers presented at the end of each chapter, and these will help you to understand more fully your own reflections and independent study. Remember, academic study will always require independent work; attending lectures will never be enough to be successful on your programme, and these activities will help to deepen your knowledge and understanding of the issues under scrutiny and give you practice at working on your own.

You might want to think about completing these activities as part of your personal development plan (PDP) or portfolio. After completing the activity, write it up in your PDP or portfolio in a section devoted to that particular skill, then look back over time to see how far you are developing. You can also do more of the activities for a key skill that you have identified a weakness in, which will help build your skill and confidence in this area.

Website for the book

In each chapter you will see a selection of words and terms highlighted in bold print where they first occur in the book. Definitions of these can be found in the glossary available on the website for this book at **www.learningmatters.co.uk/nursing**. To get to the book's webpage, click on 'Full list of nursing and midwifery titles', then click on *Introduction to Medicines Management in Nursing*. The webpage also contains a free download explaining Patient Group Directions and Non-Medical Prescribing.

Medicines Management series

This book is part of a mini-series. Other titles in this series include:

Medicines Management in Adult Nursing, Elizabeth Lawson and Dawn L. Hennefer

Medicines Management in Children's Nursing, Karen Blair

Medicines Management in Mental Health Nursing, Stanley Mutsatsa

Chapter 1
Medicines calculations
for nursing students

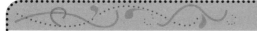

continued . . . ••

- injections including:
  - unit dose
  - sub and multiple unit dose
  - SI unit conversion.

Chapter aims

By the end of this chapter, you should be able to:

- understand the mathematical principles that underpin the accurate calculation and administration of medicines;
- discuss the consequences to the patient of receiving inaccurate dosages of medicines;
- demonstrate competence in calculating a variety of medicine dosages.

Introduction

According to the National Patient Safety Agency (NSPA, 2009), 72,482 **medication incidents** were reported in 2007. Of these, 73 per cent were reported in acute adult care and 76 per cent in acute paediatric care settings; primary care settings reported 14 per cent, while mental health settings reported 9 per cent. While the majority of such incidents resulted in little or no harm to the patients involved, 100 resulted in death or serious harm to patients. The most serious incidents occurred at the **administration stage** of medicines management (41 per cent). This report highlighted that 3,674 (5 per cent) of incidents were as a result of the wrong dose of medication being administered to patients.

An essential requirement for entry on to all pre-registration nursing programmes is the ability to demonstrate proficiency in numeracy skills. This is a requirement for all entrants by the NMC, in the interests of public protection.

While the whole process of medicines management is a responsibility of a variety of members of the **interprofessional team** (for example, doctors and pharmacists), it is generally the nurse who has the responsibility for actually giving the medicines to the patient. The administration of medicines is a task nurses perform many times each day. It is therefore essential that nurses are able to calculate medicine dosages accurately.

While only registered nurses can independently administer medicines, it is a skill that takes a lot of time, practice and experience to develop. So, as a nursing student you need to use every opportunity to practise the skills involved in the administration of medicines under the direct supervision of a registered nurse.

When performing calculations, it is important that you understand what you are doing. If you are unable to perform medicine calculations accurately and consequently give the wrong dose of medication, this could have dire consequences for your patients. Becoming familiar with some common formulas to calculate medicine dosages will help you in maintaining safe practice with medicines administration.

This chapter will help you to become familiar with some common formulas to calculate medicine dosages correctly, thereby assisting you in maintaining safe practice with the administration of medicines. First, it will look at basic mathematical principles, including **division, multiplication**, **addition**, **subtraction**, **fractions**, **decimals** and **percentages**. Next, we turn to looking at **units of weight** and **volumes** and their **equivalences**. This is important since all medications are **prescribed** and subsequently administered in a variety of weights (for example, **milligrams**) and volumes (for example, **millilitres**). Moving on from this, we will then consider the calculation of medicine dosages.

Basic mathematical principles

We utilise many basic **mathematical principles** in our daily lives, from working out our utility bills to paying for our groceries, and even to working out the interest rates on our savings or credit card. Many of us use calculators to perform such tasks. However, it is important to remember that the answers delivered by a calculator can only be as accurate as the information put into it by the user. More often than not it is human error that results in mistakes being made. In order to input correct information you still need to understand the basics of maths.

Many of the tragedies resulting from drug dosage errors could have been avoided if someone had checked the calculation again. Often it is not the numbers that are wrong, it is the amounts. Always double-check: ask yourself, is this a sensible answer? Am I quite sure the units are milligrams and not micrograms?

If you are already familiar with the basic principles of division, multiplication, addition, subtraction, fractions, decimals and percentages, you may wish to skip this section, otherwise try the activities in turn to check your understanding of these principles.

Activity 1.1

Consider the following mathematical calculations and work out the answers.

(a) You have 3 oranges, 2 bananas, 9 lemons, 3 cabbages and 12 carrots. How many pieces of citrus fruit do you have?
(b) A train carriage is carrying 5 elderly ladies, 6 adolescent males, 16 young girls and 12 middle-aged men. How many female passengers are in the train carriage?

Answers are provided at the end of the chapter.

Although these calculations are quite easy, they do require an understanding of the **denominations** being dealt with. For example, it is necessary to know that oranges and lemons are citrus fruits, while bananas, cabbages and carrots are not, and that 'ladies' and 'girls' both describe female persons. In the same way, you need to understand the context of your mathematical calculations when dealing with **medicine dosages**.

Activity 1.2   *Critical thinking*

Research a recent news story about a patient receiving the wrong dose of medicine. Think about all the possible consequences to a patient who receives the wrong dosage of a medicine. You could list them under the headings 'Too much' and 'Too little'.

An outline answer is provided at the end of the chapter.

Worked example

1 milligram + 1 milligram = 2 milligrams

and

1 milligram + 1 gram = 1001 milligrams

An amount of 1 gram is equal to 1000 milligrams. It is necessary to know that 1 gram is the same as 1000 milligrams before the sum can be accurately calculated. Medicine dosages will be covered later in this chapter.

Now answer the questions related to the following scenarios to see if you understand the principles of addition and subtraction.

Activity 1.3

A paediatric department is comprised of three wards and a day surgery unit. The wards have a bed capacity of 23, 28 and 36 inpatients respectively. The day surgery unit is able to accommodate a maximum of 17 patients at any one time.

(a) How many patients can be accommodated in the department at any given time?
(b) A total of 18 patients are due for discharge home between the three wards today. How many patients will this leave on the wards in total?
(c) The day surgery unit completed a theatre list of 16 patients this morning. Seven have since been discharged home and two patients have been transferred to the wards. How many new patients is the unit able to accommodate now?

continued overleaf . . .

continued . . .

The ward manager has £2,438 remaining in the allocated budget to spend on staff training. Staff Nurse Ahmed has requested funds to attend a one-day conference on wound management. The cost of the conference is £250. Travel costs amount to £36 for a return train ticket (standard class) and £109 for a first-class return ticket. Lunch at the conference will cost £5 and light refreshments £2.

(d) What would the total cost of attending the conference be if Staff Nurse Ahmed wishes to travel by first-class rail travel and have lunch and light refreshment in the late afternoon?

(e) What would be the remainder of the staff training budget if Staff Nurse Ahmed was to travel by standard-class rail travel and have lunch only?

(f) What would be the remainder of the budget if Staff Nurse Ahmed were to take a colleague to the conference and they each travelled by standard-class rail travel with lunch and light refreshment?

Answers are provided at the end of the chapter.

Now try the following calculations to test your understanding of the principles of multiplication.

Activity 1.4

(a) 65×36

(b) 341×5

(c) 121×7

(d) 11×11

(e) 86×64

Answers are provided at the end of the chapter.

Try the following calculations to test your understanding of the principles of division.

Activity 1.5

(a) $69 \div 3$

(b) $144 \div 12$

(c) $472 \div 8$

(d) $786 \div 6$

(e) $1100 \div 10$

Answers are provided at the end of the chapter.

If you have found any difficulty in these activities, you need to revise your basic arithmetic until you are confident in your understanding, accuracy and speed. The BBC Bitesize and the HEA Mathcentre online resources offer revision material that you can access to improve your skills. Website addresses can be found at the end of this chapter.

Using calculators

When using calculators to work out a mathematical calculation, it is vital that the correct information is inputted to the calculator and in the correct **format**. Depending on the calculator you use, it may be necessary to subtotal calculations where more than two sets of numbers are involved. This is because there is a likelihood that the wrong answer will show on the calculator, particularly with more complicated calculations, if the calculation is not subdivided into separate calculations, for example:

$3 + 4 \times 2.$

Inputting the numbers and the mathematical signs in the following stages will provide an answer of 11 when using some calculators:

Stage 1	Stage 2	Stage 3	Stage 4	Stage 5	Stage 6	Answer
3	+	4	×	2	=	11.

This answer is wrong. The correct answer is 14. To ensure you accurately calculate this sum it is necessary to input the information in the following format:

Stage 1	Stage 2	Stage 3	Stage 4	Stage 5	Stage 6	Stage 7	Stage 8	Answer
3	+	4	=	7	×	2	=	14.

Fractions

Fractions are used when dealing with numbers that are less than the whole. A fraction essentially means that it is part of a **whole number**. Like whole numbers, fractions can be added, subtracted, divided and multiplied. They can also be converted into decimals. As a nurse, you will need to know how to work with fractions, for example when you give part of an **ampoule** of medication or part of a tablet.

Understanding the terms

Fractions are expressed in the format of two numbers, one placed over another. They are separated by a dividing line. The number above the dividing line is known as a **numerator**, while the number below the line is know as a **denominator**. Here are some examples of how fractions are written:

$\frac{2}{4}$ or 2/4 (2 = numerator and 4 = denominator)

$\frac{5}{12}$ or 5/12 (5 = numerator and 12 = denominator).

If the denominator is less than the numerator, the fraction will always be greater than 1. Conversely, if the denominator is greater than the numerator, the fraction will always be less than 1.

Cancelling fractions down (simplifying fractions)

When dealing with fractions it is much easier to '**cancel down**' the numerator and the denominator; this is also known as **simplifying** fractions. This does not change the overall amount. It will usually make the calculation more straightforward and quicker to work out. In order to cancel down, the numerator and the denominator must be divided by a whole number that goes into both.

Consider the three 'bars of chocolate' below. All bars are the same size. Some of each bar has been eaten (shaded) and some remains (unshaded).

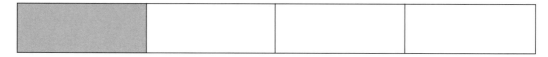

This bar has been divided into 4 equal portions. Each portion is 1/4 of the whole; 1/4 of the bar has been eaten and so 3/4 remain.

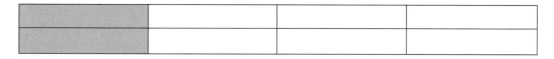

This bar has been divided into 8 equal portions. Each portion is 1/8 of the whole; 2/8 of the bar have been eaten and so 6/8 remain.

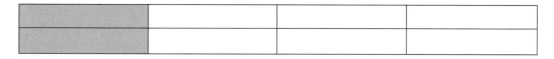

This bar has been divided into 16 equal portions. Each portion is 1/16 of the whole; 4/16 have been eaten and so 12/16 remain.

The amount of chocolate eaten from each bar is as follows:

1/4, 2/8, 4/16.

We can see that 1/4 is the same amount as 2/8 and 4/16; they are equivalent fractions.

The fraction 2/8 can be cancelled down (the numbers made smaller) by dividing both the numerator (top number) and the bottom number (denominator) by 2:

$$\frac{2 \div 2 = 1}{8 \div 2 = 4} \quad \text{and:} \quad \frac{4 \div 2 = 2}{16 \div 2 = 8}$$

$$\frac{2 \div 2 = 1}{8 \div 2 = 4}.$$

By cancelling down fractions in this way, the numbers are made smaller and easier to work with, but the overall amount or value of the number is unchanged.

Activity 1.6

Cancel down each of these fractions into its simplest form.

(a) 12/18
(b) 4/6
(c) 3/9
(d) 8/10
(e) 11/36
(f) 9/18
(g) 27/30
(h) 2/8
(i) 5/25
(j) 19/27

Answers are provided at the end of the chapter.

Adding and subtracting fractions

Provided the fractions being dealt with have the same numerator and denominator, you can add together or subtract directly.

Worked example

1/6 + 2/6 = 3/6

3/12 + 2/12 = 5/12

4/9 - 3/9 = 1/9

8/10 - 4/10 = 4/10

When adding and subtracting fractions only the numerator is changed; the denominator remains the same.

If the fractions have different denominators you will need to convert them so that they have the same denominator (see further on in this section for more details).

Adding fractions with different denominators

When adding fractions with different denominators, you should convert each fraction to an equivalent fraction, each having the same denominator. This makes them the same kind of thing, like the citrus fruits we added in Activity 1.1. In order to do this, both the numerator and denominator will need to be multiplied by the same number. This will not change the overall amount as the fraction will still be of the same value, but it will be expressed by different numbers (higher numbers); while the numbers will be different, the value of that fraction remains the same as it is an **equivalent fraction**.

Worked example

1/2 + 1/3

In this example there are many numbers that both 2 and 3 will go into: 6, 12, 18, 24 and so on. Choose the lowest number that both 2 and 3 will go into, which is 6. Multiply both parts of each fraction by the same number, so as to make the denominator of both 6:

$$\frac{1 \times 3 = 3}{2 \times 3 = 6}$$

$$\frac{1 \times 2 = 2}{3 \times 2 = 6.}$$

Now that both fractions have the same denominator it is simply a question of adding the two fractions together:

$$\frac{3 + 2 = 5}{6 + 6 = 6}$$

Subtracting fractions with different denominators

To subtract fractions you should apply the exact same principle: ensure each fraction is converted to its equivalent fraction with the same denominator. Once you have converted the fractions (if necessary), you subtract them.

Worked example

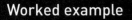

Consider what numbers 5 and 3 will both go into: 15, 30, 45 and so on. As 15 is the smallest number, convert each fraction's denominator into 15.

So by multiplying both parts of the fraction 4/5 by 3 will give a denominator of 15:

$$\frac{4 \times 3 = 12}{5 \times 3 = 15}.$$

And multiplying both parts of 2/3 by 5 will also give a denominator of 15:

$$\frac{2 \times 5 = 10}{3 \times 5 = 15}.$$

Now that both fractions have the same denominator, one fraction can be subtracted from the other:

$$\frac{12}{15} - \frac{10}{15} = \frac{2}{15}.$$

So 4/5 − 2/3 = 2/15.

There will be occasions when it is more difficult to find a lower and hence more manageable denominator that can be used for fractions.

Worked example

3/12 − 2/16

The smallest common denominator for both 12 and 16 is 48. Multiplying 12 by 4 gives 48 and multiplying 16 by 3 also gives 48:

$$\frac{3 \times 4 = 12}{12 \times 4 = 48} \quad \text{and} \quad \frac{2 \times 3 = 6}{16 \times 3 = 48}$$

These are quite bulky fractions to deal with. To make them easier to handle, you can cancel down (simplify) the fractions to begin with:

$$\frac{\cancel{3}}{\cancel{12}} = \frac{1}{4} \quad \text{and} \quad \frac{\cancel{2}}{\cancel{16}} = \frac{1}{8}.$$

So 3/12 is the same as 1/4 and 2/16 is the same as 1/8.

In order to calculate this sum write:

1/4 − 1/8 = ?

The smallest common denominator for both fractions is now 8. Therefore:

1/4 × 2 = 2/8

1/8 × 1 = 1/8.

It is now very easy to subtract one fraction from the other:

2/8 − 1/8 = 1/8.

Activity 1.7

Try the following fraction calculations.

(a) 1/5 + 2/3
(b) 4/12 + 3/9
(c) 1/2 + 2/8
(d) 2/3 − 1/6
(e) 3/8 − 1/10
(f) 1/2 − 1/3 + 2/3
(g) 3/4 + 5/8 + 1/2
(h) 6/9 − 2/18 + 1/3
(i) 4/6 − 1/3 − 1/12
(j) 9/10 + 3/20 − 4/5

Answers are provided at the end of the chapter.

Multiplying fractions

Multiplying fractions is relatively easy. All that is required is to multiply all the numerators (remember these are the numbers above the dividing line) together and then the denominators (the numbers below the dividing line).

So, for example:

$\frac{2}{7} \times \frac{9}{10}$ can be rewritten as $\frac{2 \times 9}{7 \times 10} = \frac{18}{70}$.

Worked example

$$\frac{2}{7} \times \frac{9}{10}$$

You will find it even easier to calculate if the fractions are simplified to start with. In a multiplication sum, you can cancel down the numerator of one fraction and the denominator of the other, if they are divisible by the same number. Here, the numerator 2 and denominator 10 are both divisible by 2. So

continued overleaf . . .

continued . . . .

divide the numerator '2' (in the fraction 2/7) by 2 to give a numerator of 1, and the denominator '10' (in the fraction 9/10) by 2 to give a denominator of 5.

The fraction, in its simplified form, will now look like this:

$$\frac{\cancel{2} \times 9}{7 \quad \cancel{10} 5} = \frac{1 \times 9}{7 \quad 5} = \frac{9}{35}.$$

In this example it is not possible to simplify either fraction further as there is no other common number that can be used to divide at least one other numerator and one other denominator.

It is still possible for you to multiply fractions without simplifying them first. If you prefer not to simplify them first, do remember to do so at the end. It is always good practice to express a fraction in its simplest form. So:

$$\frac{2}{7} \times \frac{9}{10} = \frac{18}{70}$$

To simplify 18/70 you should find a common divisor of both the numerator '18' and the denominator '70'. The only number (other than 1) that can be divided into both numbers is 2. So by dividing '18' and '70' by 2 you arrive at the following:

$$\frac{9\cancel{18}}{35\cancel{70}} \quad \text{The answer is} \quad \frac{9}{35}.$$

Dividing fractions

Dividing fractions is a little more complicated. This is because it involves changing the format of one fraction and then applying the principles of multiplication. So when you need to divide fractions you are not in actual fact applying any of the principles of division. When dividing fractions it is necessary to **invert** the second fraction (also called the **divisor**). Inverting in this case means turning the second fraction upside down. This means that, with the second fraction (divisor), the numerator now becomes the denominator and the denominator becomes the numerator. The two fractions are then multiplied together.

Worked example

$$\frac{3}{4} \div \frac{1}{8} \text{ becomes } \frac{3}{4} \times \frac{8}{1}$$

In this example the second fraction (divisor) 1/8 has been turned upside down (inverted). It is now expressed as 8/1.

Simplify the fractions, where possible, to make calculations easier to work out. In this example, the numbers other than 1 that can be divided into at least one numerator and one denominator, are 2 and 4. The number 4 can be divided into the denominator '4' in the fraction $\frac{3}{4}$ and the numerator '8' in the fraction $\frac{8}{1}$.

$$\frac{3}{1\!\!\!/4} \times \frac{2\!\!\!/8}{1} = \frac{3}{1} \times \frac{2}{1} = \frac{6}{1}$$

So the answer is 6.

Try the following calculations (multiplying and dividing fractions).

Activity 1.8

(a) 1/4 × 1/2
(b) 2/3 × 1/3
(c) 4/10 × 8/16
(d) 2/3 ÷ 1/4
(e) 5/9 ÷ 1/3
(f) 3/4 ÷ 2/8
(g) 1/2 × 2/8 ÷ 3/9
(h) 3/8 ÷ 4/6 × 2/3

continued overleaf . . .

continued . . .

(i) 8/9 ÷ 2/9 × 1/9

(j) 3/5 × 3/10 × 4/5

Answers are provided at the end of the chapter.

Decimals

Decimals are also known as **decimal fractions**. As with fractions, they are also used when dealing with numbers that are less than the whole. A decimal number consists of digits separated by a **decimal point**. Where the decimal point is positioned is important, as digits to the left of the decimal point represent whole numbers and so are always greater than 1. Digits to the right of the decimal point are less than 1 and are always less than 1; they are a fraction of a whole number. Each column contains numbers that are 10 times larger than those in the column to its immediate right. This means that each digit represents a different number depending on where it is positioned in relation to the decimal point.

Worked example

1206 is made up of the following values:

Whole numbers				Decimal point
Thousands	Hundreds	Tens	Units	.
1	2	0	6	.

When dealing with whole numbers only, the decimal point is usually omitted.

Consider now the following number that is made up of whole numbers and also part of a number (fraction).

Worked example

1206.456 is made up of the following values:

Whole numbers				Decimal point	Part numbers (fractions)		
Thousands	Hundreds	Tens	Units	.	Tenths	Hundredths	Thousandths
1	2	0	6	.	4	5	6

This means that 1206 is greater than .456. When dealing with part of a number only, it is necessary to place a '0' to the left of the decimal point. This is important so as not to mistake a fraction of a number with a whole number. Therefore, **.456** should be written as 0.456.

Adding and subtracting decimals

To add or subtract decimals the same principles of adding and subtracting whole numbers apply. The only extra step to consider is to place a decimal point in the answer.

Try the following calculations to retest your addition and subtraction skills. Remember to place the decimal point in the correct place in your answers.

Activity 1.9

(a) 36 + 0.006
(b) 9.65 + 3.78
(c) 432.98 + 4.78 + 3.13
(d) 98.34 − 46.32
(e) 0.002 − 0.0002
(f) 23.8 − 0.009
(g) 98 − 45.9 + 36.22
(h) 87.1 + 76.23 − 21.98
(i) 345.67 + 89.01 − 23. 45
(j) 0.008 + 0.09 − 0.005

Answers are provided at the end of the chapter.

Multiplying with decimals

To multiply using decimals it is usually easier to convert the decimal into whole numbers first. To convert a decimal to whole numbers multiply by 10, 100, 1000 and so on. It is not necessary to multiply each decimal number by the same amount. Only multiply enough to get to a whole number.

- Multiplying a decimal by 10 means that the decimal point moves one place to the right, for example $0.05 \times 10 = 0.5$
- Multiplying by 100 involves moving the decimal point two places to the right. So $0.05 \times 100 = 5$
- Multiplying the same number by 1000 requires the decimal point to move three places to the right. So $0.05 \times 1000 = 50$

When multiplying decimals together where the decimal point isn't in the same place for both decimal numbers (for example 0.05×0.6), remember to multiply by 10, 100, 1000 and so on, but only enough to get a whole number. To illustrate this let us look at the following worked example.

Worked example

Consider the calculation 0.05 x 0.6 - you can see that the decimal point is in different places for each decimal number.

To arrive at a whole number (where there are no decimal points) you will need to multiply 0.05 by 100 to reach 5 and then multiply 0.6 by 10 to reach 6. So:

0.05 x	0.6 x
100	10
5	6

Now multiply your whole numbers together: 5 x 6 = 30. But 30 is not the correct answer, because the decimal point is not in the right place.

continued overleaf . . .

continued . . .

> Count how many digits there are to the right of the decimal
> point in the two numbers that were multiplied. In the example
> above, '0.05' has two digits to the right of the decimal point and
> 0.6 has one. In total (between the two decimal numbers) there
> are three numbers to the right of the decimal point. Count the
> number of decimal places from the decimal point upwards (going
> left) in the answer. The decimal point should be placed in that
> position.
>
> This means the answer is 0.030 or 0.03. So 0.05 x 0.6 = 0.03

Rounding up or down decimals

Sometimes calculations involving decimals will provide answers with lots of numbers after the decimal point. Since it is impractical and not necessary to provide every single number after the decimal point in an answer, it will be necessary to round off answers. This is done by simply **rounding up** or **rounding down** numbers after the decimal point. Numbers below five are rounded down and numbers above five are rounded up. Depending on the calculation, it may be necessary to round off to the first, second or third decimal place. Numbers after this are small and generally insignificant; as such their value adds little if any weighting to the answer.

Table 1.1 illustrates the principles of rounding off decimal numbers.

As you can see, we have altered the values of some of these decimal numbers, by rounding up or down the digits to the right of the decimal point. The alteration in these values is so small that, generally, they do not have any real significance to the 'new' value of the decimal numbers. There

Number	One decimal place	Two decimal places	Three decimal places
106.348	106.3	106.35	106.348
0.019	0.0	0.02	0.019
3.8999	3.9	3.89	3.899

Table 1.1: Rounding off decimal numbers

are, however, some exceptions to this, particularly when dealing with very small medication dosages. This is important to note since there is a variety of medication that is manufactured, **dispensed** and administered in very small doses. Rounding off numbers in some situations may result in your patients being **underdosed** or **overdosed**.

Carry out the following calculations involving multiplying and dividing decimals. Round off each answer (where possible to two decimal places).

Activity 1.10

(a) 0.02×0.03
(b) 1.78×0.005
(c) 2.87×11.23
(d) $0.5 \div 0.005$
(e) $23.6 \div 2.4$
(f) $0.09 \div 0.003$
(g) $1.86 \times 4.22 \div 2$
(h) $89.65 \div 2.5 \times 4.66$
(i) $0.002 \times 0.03 \div 0.07$
(j) $100.01 \times 220.002 \div 3.3$

Answers are provided at the end of the chapter.

Converting fractions to decimals and decimals to fractions

It is more usual to convert fractions to decimals than the other way round, because in nursing we tend to use the **metric system** when dealing with numbers.

Electronic devices such as pumps used to administer medicine dosages to patients have metric **calibrations**, which need to be programmed to run at set **rates of infusion**. This might involve the nurse inputting whole and decimal numbers to ensure the pump runs at the correct rate to give the patient the correct medicine dosage. Medicines in general are prescribed in decimals rather than fractions. Medicine dosages will be covered later in this chapter.

Fractions to decimals

To do this simply divide the numerator by the denominator.

Worked example

$\dfrac{3}{5}$

This can be written as 3 ÷ 5 or

$5\overline{)3}$

Using the principles of division covered earlier in the chapter, you should come up with the following answer:

$5\overline{)3.0}^{\,0.6}$

So $\dfrac{3}{5}$ expressed as a decimal is 0.6

Decimals to fractions

The first step is to convert the decimal into a whole number by moving the decimal point to the right of the number.

For example, to express 0.36 as a fraction multiply 0.36 by 100 (you will need to multiply by 100 as this will turn 0.36 into the whole number '36'. So:

0.36 × 100 = 36.

The number 36 now becomes the numerator in this fraction (the number above the dividing line).

To calculate the denominator (the number below the dividing line) determine how many places the decimal point had to be moved to arrive at your 'whole number' numerator. In this example the decimal point moved two places to the right (it was multiplied by 100). Therefore the denominator for this fraction is 100.

With a numerator of 36 and a denominator of 100 the fraction will look like this:

$$\frac{36}{100.}$$

Remembering to always express a fraction in its lowest form, we now simplify the fraction.

36/100 can be simplified to 18/50, which can be further simplified to 9/25.

So 0.36 expressed as a simplified fraction is 9/25.

If we wanted to express 0.036 as a fraction, we would have to multiply by 1000 to achieve a whole number. So:

$$0.036 \times 1000 = 36$$

The number 36 becomes the numerator for this fraction. Because the decimal point in '0.036' had to be moved three times to arrive at your whole number numerator, the denominator will be 1000. The fraction will look like this:

$$\frac{36}{1000}$$

and in its simplest form it can be expressed as 9/250.

The denominator will always be expressed in values of either one-tenth, one-hundredth or one-thousandth and so on. Therefore, to work out what the denominator should be when converting decimals to fractions, you will need to multiply by either 10, 100 or 1000 and so on.

Activity 1.11

Convert the following fractions to decimals. Round off to two decimal places where possible.

(a) 1/2
(b) 2/6
(c) 4/9
(d) 8/45
(e) 11/23

Now convert the following decimals to fractions.

(f) 0.75
(g) 0.5
(h) 0.6
(i) 0.72
(j) 0.1

Answers are provided at the end of the chapter.

If you would like to undertake additional activities to further your understanding of fractions and decimals, the BBC Bitesize, HEA Mathcentre online and The Open University resources offer useful material that you can access to improve your skills. Website addresses can be found at the end of this chapter.

Percentages

Per cent means 'part of a hundred' or 'out of a hundred'. For example, 30 per cent means 30 out of 100. Percentages are useful as they can give significance to a number. For example, if it was known that 95 per cent of patients suffered **side effects** of a new medicine, this would indicate that most people had undesirable effects from the medicine (95 out of 100 people). It would probably be wise to consider asking the doctor to prescribe an alternative medication.

Percentages are also useful when making comparisons. So if, for example, 95 per cent of patients suffered side effects with a new medicine and 2 per cent of patients suffered similar effects with an alternative medicine, it would seem prudent for the alternative medicine to be the one of choice.

In nursing there will be many occasions where medicines are expressed as percentages. For example, 0.9 per cent sodium chloride, 50 per cent glucose. Later in the chapter we will look at percentages related to medicines.

In order to calculate the percentage (%) of a number, simply divide the number by 100, then multiply by the percentage value wanted.

The worked example below shows how to calculate 30 per cent of 60.

Worked example

$60 \div 100 \times 30$

$60 \div 100 = 0.6 \times 30 = 18$

So 30% of 60 = 18.

Another way to calculate the answer is to write down:

$60 = 100\%$

$0.6 = 1\%$

$0.6 \times 30 = 18$

$18 = 30\%$.

We use percentages to express the value of one number as part of another. For example, you might have 45 patients out of 416 expressing dissatisfaction with their quality of care, and you want to know how many in percentage terms were dissatisfied.

The worked example below shows how to calculate what percentage 45 is of 416.

Worked example

$45 \div 416 = 0.108$

To express the answer 0.108 as a percentage you will need to multiply by 100:

$0.108 \times 100 = 10.8$

Therefore, 45 out of 416 expressed as a percentage is 10.8 per cent.

Another way to calculate the percentage would be to write:

$416 = 100\%$

$$1\% = \frac{100}{416}$$

So:

$$
\begin{array}{r}
0.24 \\
416\overline{)100\ 0} \\
83\ 2 \\
\hline
16\ 80 \\
16\ 64 \\
\hline
16
\end{array}
$$

This means that 1 per cent is equivalent to 0.24 (out of the total of 416). So once again:

$0.24 \times 45 = 10.8.$

Activity 1.12

Try the following calculations (round off answers to the nearest whole number).

(a) 10% of 600
(b) 33.25% of 89
(c) 12% of 106
(d) 99% of 150
(e) 11% of 298

Now express the following values as a percentage (again round off answers to the nearest whole percentage point).

(f) 45 out of 98
(g) 765 out of 770
(h) 3 out of 10
(i) 44 out of 765
(j) 20 out of 100

Answers are provided at the end of the chapter.

If you would like to undertake additional activities to further your understanding of percentages, the BBC Bitesize, HEA Mathcentre online and The Open University resources offer useful material that you can access to improve your skills. Website addresses can be found at the end of this chapter.

Units and equivalences: units of weight and volume

Medicines, be they in tablet, liquid or powder form, have their **strength** expressed in units of weight or volume.

- Tablets and powder forms of medication are generally expressed in terms of weight (for example, **micrograms**, milligrams, grams).
- Liquids are generally expressed in terms of volume (for example, millilitres, **litres**). They can also be expressed in **moles** or **millimoles**.

It is important to be familiar with how medicine strengths are expressed. It is also vital to know what their equivalences (alternative measurements) are. This is necessary because, many times a day, nurses need to administer to patients prescribed medicines where the dosage (strength) is prescribed in a different measurement from that supplied by the pharmacy department.

It is necessary to know the common units of strength, their abbreviations and their equivalences. These are detailed in Table 1.2.

Please note that it is recommended that micrograms and nanograms should not be abbreviated – that is, using the symbols 'mcg' and 'ng' (BNF, 2010). However, there may be occasions when you see these abbreviations in books, journal articles or even on patients'

Unit	Abbreviation	Equivalent	Abbreviation
1 **kilogram**	kg	1000 grams	g
1 gram	g	1000 milligrams	mg
1 milligram	mg	1000 micrograms	mcg
1 microgram	mcg	1000 **nanograms**	ng
1 litre	l or L	1000 millilitres	ml
1 mole	mol	1000 millimoles	mmol
1 millimole	mmol	1000 **micromoles**	mcmol

Table 1.2: Metric units and their equivalents

prescriptions. You must always follow your Trust/Employer and University policies regarding the approved abbreviations that you are allowed to use. We have used these abbreviations in this chapter to save space. Great care should be taken not to confuse ng (nanograms) with mcg (micrograms) as this can lead to errors.

It is rare in adult patients to have medicines prescribed in nanograms (ng) or micromoles (mcmol), but it is more common with children because of the smaller dosages required to bring about the **desired effect**. Note that when dealing with plurals in an abbreviation, the 's' is not included (write 2mg and not 2mgs).

Converting units

Each unit of strength differs from the adjacent one by a factor of 100. This means that to convert one strength to another you should multiply or divide by 1000. So, to express strength in a lower unit of measurement, multiply by 1000 and to express strength in a higher one, divide by 1000. When carrying out medicine calculations it is always easier and hence safer to work in whole numbers. For example, when giving 0.5 litres of a medication, convert this into millilitres to get a whole number:

$0.5 \times 1000 = 500$ ml.

Activity 1.13

Convert the following. Remember to include the correct unit in your answers.

(a) 3 milligrams into micrograms
(b) 500 micrograms into milligrams
(c) 10 grams into milligrams
(d) 1 gram into milligrams
(e) 3000 nanograms into micrograms

continued overleaf . . .

continued . . .

(f) 0.5 milligrams into micrograms
(g) 0.75 grams into milligrams
(h) 50 micrograms into nanograms
(i) 0.25 litres into millilitres
(j) 3 moles into millimoles

Answers are provided at the end of the chapter.

It is vitally important to move the decimal point the correct number of places (three places in this case) to prevent administering an incorrect dose to the patient.

Medicine concentrations or strengths

Medications are manufactured in many formats, including tablet, liquid, powder, spray and cream formats. There are several ways of expressing the concentration or strength of a medicine present in a medication preparation. This applies to medicines for **oral**, **topical** (**transdermal**), **inhalation**, **sublingual**, **subcutaneous**, **intramuscular** and **intravenous** use (these routes will be explained in more detail in Chapter 3). When dealing with medicines in their liquid form, the most common way is to state milligrams (mg) of the medicine per millilitre (ml), expressed as mg/ml. The strength of other medicines might be expressed as micrograms (mcg) per millilitre (ml) or nanograms (ng) per millilitre (ml). For example, the pharmacist stocks metoclopramide 5mg/ml and digoxin 100mcg/ml.

Medicine prescriptions should state the strength of the medicine to be given rather than the volume of the liquid or the number of tablets. This is because different strengths can be manufactured for the same medicine. For example, flucloxacillin, for oral use, is manufactured in 250mg and 500mg capsules. It is also manufactured in syrup form as 125mg/5ml and 250mg/5ml.

Examples of how prescriptions should be written can be seen on the **prescription chart** in Figure 1.1.

Another way to express concentrations of medicines is by **percentage concentration**. Percentage concentration means the amount of the active drug in 100 parts of the product. This is normally used when a solid has been dissolved in liquid. It refers to the number of grams (solid drug by weight) that have been dissolved in 100ml (volume of liquid). The abbreviated term used to express the percentage concentration is '% w/v'. The 'w' refers to the weight of the drug (for example 10mg) and the 'v' refers to the volume of liquid it has been dissolved in (this will always be 100ml).

The worked example on p31 shows how to express the percentage concentration of a drug that has been dissolved in liquid.

SURNAME	FORENAME	DATE OF BIRTH	PATIENT IDENTIFICATION NUMBER	ALLERGIES
Bridges	Beryl	01/11/1930	143986	None known

HEIGHT	WEIGHT	CONSULTANT	SPECIAL DIETARY REQUIREMENTS	
1.65m	65kg	Langley	None	

ONCE ONLY DRUGS/VARIABLE DOSE PRESCRIPTIONS

Date	Drug	Dose	Route	Prescriber's signature	Administered by	Date and time	Pharmacy
29/09/10	Clexane	20mg	S.C	R. Wright	M. Arkah	29/09/10 at 06.00	

REGULAR PRESCRIPTIONS

	Time	Date										
Drug Digoxin	08.00											
Route O / Dose 125mcg / Start Date 29/09/10 / End Date 03/10/10												
Prescriber's Signature R. Wright / Pharmacy												
Drug Lactulose	08.00											
Route O / Dose 10ml / Start Date 29/09/10 / End Date 03/10/10												
Prescriber's Signature R. Wright / Pharmacy	20.00											
Drug Amoxicillin	06.00											
Route I.V / Dose 500mg / Start Date 29/09/10 / End Date 03/10/10	14.00											
Prescriber's Signature R. Wright / Pharmacy	22.00											
Drug Paracetamol	06.00											
Route P.R / Dose 1g / Start Date 29/09/10 / End Date 03/10/10	12.00 18.00											
Prescriber's Signature R. Wright / Pharmacy	24.00											

Figure 1.1: Prescription chart

Worked example

% w/v = grams in 100 ml

So 3 per cent w/v means 3g of a drug in 100ml of liquid.

Percentage concentrations may also be expressed as the number of grams of a drug in 100g. This means that a drug has been added to another solid product. So, to express the percentage concentration of a drug that has been added to another solid product, the expression '% w/w' is used, meaning weight per weight or the number of grams in 100g.

Worked example

3 per cent w/w means 3g of drug in 100g of a solid product.

Finally, another way to express percentage concentrations is where a specific volume (for example millilitres) of a medicine has been added to another liquid product. The percentage concentration is expressed as the liquid amount of the medicine added to another liquid product. This can be written as '% v/v' meaning volume per volume or the number of millilitres in 100ml.

Worked example

3 per cent v/v means 3ml of a drug in 100ml of another liquid product.

Activity 1.14

Consider the following medicine concentrations.

Your patient has been prescribed oramorph 5mg. In **stock** you have the following concentrations of oramorph:

10mg in 5ml
5mg in 10ml
20mg in 5ml.

continued overleaf . . .

continued . . . ••

(a) How many millilitres (ml) of each of the above concentrations of oramorph would you give?

(b) If the prescription read that you should administer 5ml of oramorph, what would you do?

(c) Consider and list the possible consequences to your patient for each of the amounts of the medication had you given them to your patient in answer (b). (You should assume that the intended dose the patient should have is oramorph 5mg.)

Answers are provided at the end of the chapter.

Calculation of medicine dosages

Dispensing and administering medicines in tablet, capsule or liquid form is a regular task for nurses. To ensure the correct amount of a medicine is given to each patient, you have to apply the basic principles of maths in order to calculate the correct dosage. You also need to be competent and feel confident in your ability to convert units of weight and volume into their equivalences. (This is one of the most common sources of drug dose errors.)

Medicines to be administered in solid form

For medicines to be administered in their solid form, such as tablets or capsules, the basic formula to use for calculating the amount of a medicine to be given is:

$$\frac{\text{What you want}}{\text{What you've got}} \quad \text{or} \quad \frac{\text{Prescribed dose}}{\text{Stock dosage (what's in the bottle)}}$$

This means that the prescribed dosage needs to be divided by the stock dosage that is available.

Worked example

If a patient is prescribed thyroxine 250mcg and the stock dosage (strength of medication available) is 125mcg, then 2 tablets would need to be given:

$$\frac{\text{Thyroxine } 250\text{mcg}}{\text{Thyroxine } 125\text{mcg}} = 2 \text{ tablets}$$

This is a relatively easy calculation since the prescribed dosage and the stock dosage are in the same unit of strength, in this case micrograms (mcg).

When the prescribed dosage and the stock dosage are of different strengths, it is necessary to convert one of them into the same strength, but still maintain their unit equivalence. This means that the dosage calculation should be worked out in the same unit. This is where **dosage conversion** is necessary. It is best practice to try to avoid working with decimal points as serious errors can occur. Imagine the consequences of putting a decimal point in the wrong place. The patient could end up with ten, a hundred or even a thousand times too much of the medication. (We hear about the resulting tragedies too often on the news.)

Consider the following example of how to carry out dosage conversions when dealing with prescribed and stock dosages in differing units of strength.

Worked example

A patient is prescribed digoxin 0.25mg. The stock is 125mcg tablets. It is better and safer to convert the prescription dosage in this case as it eliminates the need for working with decimal points. Therefore, to work out how many tablets to give the patient, convert the prescribed dose of 0.25mg (milligrams) into micrograms (mcg). To remind yourself of equivalences, refer back to the section on units and equivalences on pp27-9.

So, 0.250 x 1000 = 250mcg.

Then divide 250mcg by the stock dosage available (125mcg):

250mcg ÷ 125mcg = 2 tablets.

Consider the same patient again. The patient is still prescribed digoxin 0.25mg. This time, the stock dosage is 62.5mcg. After converting the prescribed dosage to micrograms, the patient would require 4×62.5mcg tablets.

Although it is possible to give either combination of tablets, such as 2×125mcg tablets or 4×62.5mcg tablets, since both total the same amount, it is good practice to give the lowest possible number of tablets. Therefore in this case, the 125mcg tablets should be dispensed.

Medicines to be administered in liquid form

When calculating the amount of a medicine to give in liquid form the following formula can be used:

$$\frac{\text{What you want}}{\text{What you've got}} \times \text{the volume it is in}$$

or

$$\frac{\text{Prescribed dose}}{\text{Stock dosage (what's in the bottle)}} \times \text{the volume of the stock dosage}$$

Consider the following prescription.

Worked example

A patient has been prescribed haloperidol 2mg via the intramuscular (IM) route. The stock dosage is 5mg/ml. Refer back to pp29-32 in the section titled 'Medicine concentrations or strengths' if necessary.

To calculate the correct amount of haloperidol to administer:

$$\frac{2mg \times 1ml}{5mg} = \frac{2 \times 1}{5}$$

Divide 5mg into 2mg. This gives 0.4 mg. Then multiply 0.4mg by 1.

$$0.4mg \times 1 = 0.4ml$$

The patient would need to be administered 0.4ml of haloperidol.

Another sensible rule to follow when calculating medicine dosages is to be mindful if your answer looks unlikely, for instance if it requires you to administer a large number of tablets or volumes of liquid. It is always useful to double-check a calculation if this happens, in case the calculation is inaccurate. Similarly, if a calculation suggests a very small amount of liquid dosage or splitting a tablet it is worthwhile rechecking the calculation.

Medicine dosages based on body weight and body surface area

There will be many times when medicine dosages have to be administered according to the weight of the patient, particularly for children, or the **body surface area** (**BSA**). Some medicine dosages are also calculated to take into account other parameters, such as **renal function** or age.

Medicine dosages based on body weight

Medicine dosages prescribed relative to body weight are always calculated according to the patient's weight in kilograms (kg). For example, the medicine will be prescribed as mg per kg, mcg per kg, ng per kg and so on. In order to determine the correct dosage, multiply the prescribed dosage by the patient's body weight in kilograms. For example: a patient is prescribed dexamethasone 150mcg/kg. He weighs 8kg. The dose to be given is shown in the worked example below.

Worked example

150mcg x 8 = 1200mcg or 1.2mg.

Medicine dosages based on body surface area

The dosage of some medicines may be calculated on BSA, in square metres (m^2). BSA is calculated for certain medicines, such as **cytotoxic medicines** (those used to treat cancer), where there is very little difference between an effective and a **toxic dosage**. In other words, if too much of a medicine is administered (this extra amount may be very small) it may produce toxic rather than **therapeutic effects**. A medicine dosage based on BSA is much safer because many **physiological factors** are linked to BSA, for example the blood flow to the kidneys and the liver, two of the major body organs associated with the **metabolism** and **excretion** of medicines (see Chapter 3 for further information on metabolism and excretion of medicines). To determine the patient's BSA, their height and weight must be known. The BSA can be calculated using the following formula devised by Mosteller (1987):

$$m^2 \text{ (BSA)} = \sqrt{\frac{\text{height (cm)} \times \text{weight (kg)}}{3600}}$$

Case study

Your patient Jenny Glendenning is to be prescribed a medicine based on her BSA. She is 90cm in height and weighs 13.2kg. You have to calculate Jenny's body surface area.

Using the formula above, these parameters are placed as follows:

$$BSA = \sqrt{\frac{90 \times 13.2}{3600}} = \frac{1188}{3600} = 0.33$$

*The next step is to find the **square root** ($\sqrt{}$) of 0.33. This is 0.574 m^2. It is easier and much quicker to work this out with a calculator using the following steps:*

- *Input '0.33'.*
- *Then press the square root key (marked with the sign '$\sqrt{}$').*
- *Finally, press the equal or total key (marked with the sign '=').*

You should get the result that Jenny's BSA is 0.574 m^2.

Do ask a colleague to check your calculation.

There are many formulas that can be used to calculate the BSA; the Mosteller formula is a relatively quick and simple one to use.

You may also come across the use of a **nomogram** to obtain a BSA. A nomogram is a graphical representation of numerical relationships. Parameters are plotted on each graph. A straight line is then drawn through each plotted parameter (height and weight). Where the line intersects with the BSA column, this indicates the body surface area. A nomogram will only provide an estimate of the BSA.

The next case study gives an example of a medicine prescription based on BSA.

Case study

Your patient Wesley Grimes is prescribed 75mg/m^2 of doxorubicin. He has a BSA of 1.7m^2.

To calculate how much of the medicine Wesley should have, multiply the required dosage by the BSA.

75 $\times$ 1.7 = 127.5

Wesley requires 127.5mg of doxorubicin.

Try the following calculations related to medicine dosages.

Activity 1.15

A prescription reads to administer:

(a) 400mg of ibuprofen via the oral route. The stock dosage is 200mg. How many tablets should be given?

(b) 125mg of paracetamol via the oral route. The stock dosage is in a liquid form (suspension) of 500mg/10ml. How many millilitres should be given?

(c) 40mg of flupentixol decanoate via the intramuscular route. The stock dosage is 20mg/ml. How many millilitres should be given?

(d) 0.625mg of digoxin via the oral route. There are two stock dosages available, 500mcg tablets and 62.5 mcg tablets. What is the best combination of tablets to give?

(e) 62.5mg of amoxicillin via the oral route. The stock dosage is in a **suspension** of 125mg/5ml. How many millilitres should be given?

(f) Furosemide 0.5mg/kg via the oral route. The patient weighs 15kg. How many milligrams should be given?

(g) Gentamicin 4mg/kg via the intramuscular route. The patient weighs 62kg. The stock dosage is 40mg/ml. How many milligrams should be given?

(h) Gentamicin 4mg/kg via the intramuscular route. The patient weighs 62kg. The stock dosage is 40mg/ml. The patient has been prescribed the dosage, divided into three doses per day. How many millilitres should be given each time it is due?

(i) Prednisolone 60mg/m^2 via the oral route. The patient has a BSA of 0.45m^2. How many milligrams should be given?

(j) Desmopressin 2000ng via the subcutaneous route. The stock dosage is 4mcg/ml. How many micrograms and millilitres should be given?

Answers are provided at the end of the chapter.

Calculating intravenous infusion rates

Administering intravenous (IV) fluids is one of the most common therapeutic techniques used in hospitals. It is used for a variety of reasons, such as correcting **fluid and electrolyte imbalances** or as a **medium** for the administration of medicines. There are three stages to working out the **rate** at which IV fluids are given. A rate is an amount per unit of time.

- Stage 1: How many millilitres per hour need to be given?
- Stage 2: How many millilitres per minute need to be given?
- Stage 3: How many drops per minute need to be given?

Intravenous fluids are administered using a piece of equipment called a **giving set**, also called an **administration set**. A giving set is simply a long piece of tubing that allows the fluid to drain from the bag containing the intravenous fluid into the patient via a **cannula** (a small plastic tube inserted into the patient's vein; the plural is cannulae). There are several different types of giving sets and the number of drops required to deliver 1ml of fluid will vary with each type of giving set.

A **standard giving set** for an infusion to be administered by gravity, and for administering an **aqueous solution** or **crystalloid** (such as normal saline), will be capable of holding 20 drops of fluid per millilitre.

A standard giving set for an infusion to be administered by gravity and for administering a **colloid** (such as blood, blood products or plasma expanding agents) will be capable of holding 15 drops of fluid per millilitre. This is because these products have a more **viscous**, or thicker, consistency.

Another giving set that can be used is a **microdrop giving set** (commonly known as a **burette** or a **paediatric giving set**). Such a set can hold 60 drops per millilitre of crystalloid solutions.

Whenever possible, intravenous infusions (IVIs) should be administered via an **infusion pump**, which provides exact control over the rate that the fluid is running. Like all such machines, its accuracy depends on the correct information being inputted.

Consider a typical IVI prescription in the case study below.

Case study

Your patient Rubina Kapour is prescribed 1 litre of normal saline to be administered over 8 hours.

Using the stages described above:

Stage 1:   1 litre = 1000 millilitres

1000 ÷ 8 = 125

Therefore Rubina requires 125ml of normal saline per hour.

Stage 2:   125ml ÷ 60 seconds = 2.08ml per minute. This means Rubina needs to receive 2.08ml of normal saline per minute.

To be able to progress to Stage 3 the number of drops of fluid per millilitre needs to be calculated.

Since we are infusing a crystalloid we will be using a standard giving set that is capable of holding 20 drops of fluid per ml. So:

Stage 3:   Multiply millilitres per minute by drops per millilitre to arrive at how many drops per minute the infusion should be set to run at:

2.08 × 20 = 41.6 = 42 drops per minute.

Rubina's infusion should run at 42 drops per minute.

continued overleaf . . .

continued . . . •••

Put simply, the formula to calculate IVI drip rates is:

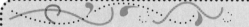

$$\frac{\textit{Drops per ml of the giving set} \times \textit{amount in ml to be infused}}{\textit{Total infusion time in minutes}}$$

Activity 1.16

Assuming that standard giving sets are being used, calculate the following. Give your answers in ml/hr and also drops per minute and round your answers to the nearest whole number.

(a) 500ml of 5% dextrose over 6 hours

(b) 350ml of blood over 3 hours

(c) 300ml of normal saline over 6 hours (using a standard paediatric giving set that is capable of holding 60 drops per ml)

(d) 1 litre of gelofusine over 5 hours

(e) 600ml of blood over 4 hours

(f) 1.2 litres of 0.9% sodium chloride over 8 hours

(g) 100ml of dextrose saline over 2 hours

(h) 45ml of 5% dextrose over 1 hour

(i) 2.5 litres of 0.9% sodium chloride over 12 hours

(j) 400ml of dextrose saline over 90 minutes

Answers are provided at the end of the chapter.

Chapter summary

This chapter has helped you check your understanding of the basic mathematical principles of addition, subtraction, multiplication and division. It has then looked at the principles of dealing with fractions, decimals and percentages. Units, equivalences and medicine concentrations have also been reviewed in this chapter. Only once you have understood all these principles should you progress to applying them to medicines administration. Medicine dosage calculations, including those based on patient parameters (for example, height and weight measurements), have been considered. Finally, calculating intravenous infusion rates has been explored. By working through the variety of mathematical exercises, you should be able to self-assess your abilities with all of the above. Completion of these activities will assist you in achieving the necessary proficiency for entry into your field of practice programme.

Activities: brief outline answers

Activity 1.1 (page 6)

12 pieces of citrus fruit
21 female passengers

Activity 1.2 (page 7)

If the patient is given too much of a medication it could cause them physical harm. They may be overdosed on the medication, which may cause undesirable side effects. This could lead to irreversible damage to an organ or a body system and in some cases could lead to the untimely death of a patient. If the patient is given too small a dose it will cause the body to be depleted of the medication and consequently the patient, an organ or a body system may be left untreated. It may also cause the patient psychological harm. It may also lead to mistrust of nursing staff and other healthcare professionals by the patient. Once this trust is broken it can be difficult to regain.

Activity 1.3 (page 7)

(a) 104
(b) 69
(c) 10
(d) £366
(e) £2147
(f) £1852

Activity 1.4 (page 8)

(a) 2340
(b) 1705
(c) 847
(d) 121
(e) 5504

Activity 1.5 (page 8)

(a) 23
(b) 12
(c) 59
(d) 131
(e) 110

Activity 1.6 (page 11)

(a) 2/3
(b) 2/3
(c) 1/3
(d) 4/5
(e) 11/36
(f) 1/2
(g) 9/10
(h) 1/4

(i)   1/5
(j)   19/27

Activity 1.7 (page 15)

(a)   13/15
(b)   2/3
(c)   3/4
(d)   1/2
(e)   11/40
(f)   5/6
(g)   15/8 or 1 7/8
(h)   8/9
(i)   1/4
(j)   1/4

Activity 1.8 (page 17)

(a)   1/8
(b)   1/3
(c)   1/5
(d)   2 2/3
(e)   1 2/3
(f)   3
(g)   3/8
(h)   3/8
(i)   4/9
(j)   18/125

Activity 1.9 (page 19)

(a)   36.006
(b)   13.43
(c)   440.89
(d)   52.02
(e)   0.0018
(f)   23.791
(g)   88.32
(h)   141.35
(i)   411.23
(j)   0.093

Activity 1.10 (page 22)

(a)   0
(b)   0.01
(c)   32.23
(d)   100
(e)   9.83
(f)   30
(g)   3.92
(h)   167.11
(i)   0
(j)   6667.39

Activity 1.11 (page 24)

(a) 0.5
(b) 0.33
(c) 0.44
(d) 0.18
(e) 0.48
(f) 3/4
(g) 1/2
(h) 2/3
(i) 18/25
(j) 1/10

Activity 1.12 (page 27)

(a) 60
(b) 29 or 30
(c) 13
(d) 148
(e) 33
(f) 46%
(g) 99%
(h) 30%
(i) 6%
(j) 20%

Activity 1.13 (page 28)

(a) 3000mcg
(b) 0.5mg
(c) 10000mg
(d) 1000mg
(e) 3mcg
(f) 500mcg
(g) 750mg
(h) 50000ng
(i) 250ml
(j) 3000mmol

Activity 1.14 (pages 31–2)

(a) 2.5ml, 10ml, 1.25ml.
(b) You should not dispense this medicine. The prescription is incorrect as it states only volume. The strength of the medicine must be included in the prescription. You should ask the doctor to change the prescription to state the strength in which the medicine should be administered.
(c) If 10mg is administered the patient will receive twice the intended dose. This is an overdose and may lead to undesirable side effects and complications for the patient.

   If 2.5mg is administered the patient will receive half the intended dose. This is an underdose and may not be effective in controlling or relieving the patient's condition (in this case, pain).

   If 20mg is administered the patient will receive four times the intended dose. This is an overdose and it is likely that this will lead to undesirable side effects and serious complications for the patient.

Activity 1.15 (page 37)

(a) 2 tablets
(b) 2.5ml

(c) 2ml

(d) 1 × 500mcg tablet, 2 × 62.5mcg tablet

(e) 2.5ml

(f) 7.5mg

(g) 248mg

(h) 2.06ml

(i) 27mg

(j) 2mcg, 0.5ml

Activity 1.16 (page 39)

(a) 83ml/hr, 28 drops per minute

(b) 117ml/hr, 29 drops per minute

(c) 50ml/hr, 50 drops per minute

(d) 200ml/hr, 50 drops per minute (gelofusine is a plasma expanding agent so you would use a giving set capable of holding 15 drops of fluid per millilitre)

(e) 150ml/hr, 37 drops per minute

(f) 150ml/hr, 50 drops per minute

(g) 50ml/hr, 17 drops per minute

(h) 45ml/hr, 15 drops per minute

(i) 208ml/hr, 69 drops per minute

(j) 266ml/hr, 89 drops per minute

Knowledge review

Now that you've worked through the chapter, how would you rate your knowledge of the following topics?

	Good	Adequate	Poor
The basic mathematical principles of: 1. Addition 2. Subtraction 3. Multiplication 4. Division 5. Adding and subtracting fractions 6. Multiplying and dividing fractions 7. Adding and subtracting decimals 8. Multiplying and dividing decimals 9. Converting fractions to decimals 10. Converting decimals to fractions 11. Calculating percentages			
Formulas to calculate: 1. Units and their equivalences 2. Medicine dosages based on strength 3. Medicine dosages based on volume 4. Medicine dosages based on body weight 5. Medicine dosages based on BSA 6. Intravenous infusion rates			

Where you're not confident in your knowledge of a topic, what will you do next?

Further reading

Lapham, L and Agar, H (2009) *Drug Calculations for Nurses: A step by step approach*, 3rd edition. London: Hodder Arnold.

This is an easy-to-read book explaining the practical application of the mathematical principles needed for accurate medicine calculations.

National Patient Safety Agency (NPSA) (2009) *Safety in Doses: Improving the use of medicines in the NHS.* London: National Patient Safety Agency.

This is a detailed review by the NPSA outlining medication incidents reported in 2007 in NHS care settings.

Starkings, S and Krause, L (2010) *Passing Calculations Tests for Nursing Students.* Exeter: Learning Matters.

This book helps new nursing students succeed first time in medicines calculations tests, and get calculations right in practice. It takes the fear out of maths, even for those who find it a struggle, through clear step-by-step explanations and lively examples.

Useful websites

http://labspace.open.ac.uk

The Open University (OU) OpenLearn website gives free access to learning materials from higher education courses. To access this site registration is required, but it is free of charge. The following are relevant to your studies here:

Numbers, units and arithmetic: **http://labspace.open.ac.uk/course/view.php?id=3434**

Rounding and estimation: **http://labspace.open.ac.uk/course/view.php?id=3586**

www.bbc.co.uk/schools/ks2bitesize/maths/number

www.bbc.co.uk/schools/gcsebitesize/maths/number

The BBC Bitesize online resources offer revision material that you can use to enhance your understanding of basic mathematical principles. The web pages above are free of charge and can help you with the arithmetic required for this chapter.

www.bnf.org/bnf

This is the home of the online *British National Formulary* (BNF), where information on clinical conditions, medicines and their preparations can be reviewed. Please note that user registration is required, although this is free of charge.

www.bnfc.org/bnfc

This gives access to the online BNF for children, where information on clinical conditions, medicines and their preparations can be reviewed. Please note that user registration is required, although this is free of charge.

www.mathcentre.ac.uk/students.php/health/arithmetic

Another free useful online resource is the Higher Education Academy Centre for Excellence in Teaching and Learning Mathcentre, which offers quick reference guides, practice and revision materials, video tutorials, workbooks and online practice exercises on many branches of mathematics.

www.npsa.nhs.uk/nrls

This site, set up by the NPSA, deals with the reporting of untoward incidents, including medication incidents, that have occurred in NHS care settings.

Chapter 2
Legal and professional issues in medicines management

Introduction

This chapter sets out the legal, regulatory, professional and ethical contexts in which nurses are empowered to administer medication to patients. It will introduce you to the relevant law and government regulations related to the control of medicines in hospital and the community in the United Kingdom, and will detail the role and function of the Nursing and Midwifery Council (NMC) guidance in the management of medicines by nurses. Ethical considerations will also be addressed. Having knowledge of the law and professional guidance will prepare you for specific modules on your chosen field of practice, where you will learn more about medicines management related to your field. In this chapter you will also learn where you can find up-to-date information about all kinds of medicines. In these respects you will be able to acquire the competencies and essential skills detailed above. Other NMC competencies and Essential Skills Clusters are also relevant to medicines management, but are not specifically addressed in this chapter – you can find these in other chapters.

The administration of medicines is an important function of the role of the registered nurse and for many aspiring nurses this is the key function that sets the qualified nurse apart from students and other health professionals. This function includes a responsibility to service users, the patient or client, the public and to the law as well as to the nursing profession, and must be discharged in a safe and competent manner within the law and the professional framework of the nursing profession. As a student nurse in training for the NMC register, you are not allowed to give any medicine to a service user, patient or client unless you are assisting a registered nurse, and you must be actively supervised in this process at all times. Once you enter the NMC register, you take on the responsibility of a registered nurse and all the professional and ethical principles that this entails, and you must prepare for that role while you are a student, so that you can act independently in the future. The law and associated regulations and professional guidance exist to help you in discharging your responsibilities. These laws exist to regulate and/or control everything relating to medicines.

Medicines legislation and nursing practice

What is a medicine?

Historically, humans have made use of all kinds of substances to help them deal with bodily ailments, including substances derived from plants, animals, metals and minerals. Ancient Greek, Egyptian, Chinese and Arab cultures have all left evidence of the way they used rudimentary pharmacological compounds for the purpose of healing. It was not until late in the nineteenth and early in the twentieth centuries that the modern science of pharmacology emerged and, over the course of the last century, pharmacology has become a sophisticated science that uses modern scientific methods to produce better targeted medications. With this emergence came the need for control and regulation of medicines and medicinal products. The Medicines Act 1968 (HMSO, 1968) is the basis on which medicines are manufactured, tested and quality controlled before they reach the patient. While a detailed knowledge of the Act and subsequent amendments and associated regulations is not necessary, every nurse needs a fundamental knowledge of those aspects of the law that control medicines. This Act and other relevant legislation and its implications will now be discussed.

The Medicines Act 1968

This Act sets out the legislation that controls the manufacture, importation, exportation and supply of all medicinal products. Drugs, or medicines, liable to abuse and misuse are controlled by the Misuse of Drugs Act 1971 (HMSO, 1971), hence the use of the term **controlled drugs** (CDs). A medicine is defined by the Medicines Act as being *a substance or article, or an ingredient that is used for a medicinal purpose*; a medicinal purpose is defined as:

- the treatment and prevention of disease;
- diagnosing or ascertaining the existence, degree or extent of a physiological condition;
- contraception;
- inducing anaesthesia;
- otherwise preventing or interfering with the normal operation of a physiological function.

It can be seen from this list that there is potentially a large number of substances that can be classified as medicines.

Categories of medicines

There are three categories of medicines defined under the Act.

General sales list (GSL) medicines

These are medicines that can be sold in a general store, such as a supermarket or corner shop, as well as being available for sale in a pharmacy (chemist's shop). A huge number of medicines come into this category. Most people would have some in their own homes, and it would not be uncommon for a patient to have some with them when admitted to hospital. Examples of these would be mild analgesics such as paracetamol tablets, aspirin tablets or ibuprofen gel; medicines for constipation such as senna tablets; creams for haemorrhoids ('piles'); calamine lotion for skin irritation; indigestion remedies; and cough mixtures. There are no general restrictions on their sale, but there is nevertheless potential for abuse or misuse as with any medicinal product. For example, the Medicines and Healthcare products Regulatory Agency (MHRA) provides guidance for shopkeepers in respect of some analgesic medications such as paracetamol, which if taken in large amounts can cause liver damage, and the MHRA discourages multiple sales and multi-buy promotions for these analgesics. Many shopkeepers set up their tills so that, for example, no more that 32 tablets of paracetamol can be sold in one transaction.

Pharmacy-only (P) medicines

These are medicines that can only be sold from a pharmacy and are not available on open shelves for customers to help themselves. These medicines are sold under the control of a pharmacist, who must be present when the sale is made. No definitive list is available, but these medicines can be identified by the letter 'P' on the packaging. The pharmacist may ask a customer questions to ascertain if what they are requesting is appropriate for their symptoms.

Prescription-only medicines (POMs)

These are medicines that can only be sold or supplied on the presentation of a **prescription** from a medical or dental practitioner or a nurse prescriber. There are three classes of prescription-only medicines:

- those that contain listed substances;
- those containing a drug controlled by the Misuse of Drugs Act 1971;
- medicinal products that are for **parenteral** use, i.e. injectable substances.

These are the legal categories of medicines controlled by the 1968 Act (HMSO, 1968). However, when a person is a patient in hospital, all medicines, whatever their legal category, must be prescribed by a medical, dental or nurse prescriber. The Act states that no one other than a registered doctor, dentist or **supplementary prescriber**, or someone acting in accordance with the instructions of such a practitioner, may administer a POM to a person other than themselves.

Most other countries have similar medicines legislation. All amendments to the United Kingdom Medicines Act must now comply with European (EU) Law.

Activity 2.1   *Evidence-based practice and research*

Look at the following list of medicines. Decide which category each medicine falls under. You may wish to compile a table for your answer using the following headings: GSL, P and POM. You may need to refer to the BNF to help you with this activity.

Codeine phosphate

Ibuprofen

Paracetamol

Piriton

Ranitidine

Salbutamol

Bacillus Calmette-Guerin (BCG) vaccine

Chloramphenicol eye drops

Bonjela

An outline answer is provided at the end of the chapter.

The Misuse of Drugs Act 1971

This is an important piece of legislation that controls drugs that are liable to abuse and misuse (HMSO, 1971). It is the Act under which people can be prosecuted for the illegal manufacture, supply and possession of substances such as diamorphine (heroin), cocaine, cannabis, ecstasy and amphetamines. The Act defines three **classes** of drugs according to how harmful they are perceived to be if they are abused, with drugs in class A being identified as the most harmful, drugs in Class B less harmful and drugs in Class C the least harmful (see Table 2.1). This in no way implies that any drug not controlled by the Misuse of Drugs Act is not harmful, as all drugs have the potential to cause harm if not used properly. Drugs can be added to the list as required,

Class	Examples of drugs in each class
Class A: the most harmful	Ecstasy, LSD, heroin, cocaine, magic mushrooms, methylamphetamine (crystal meth), injectable amphetamines.
Class B: an intermediate category	Cannabis, amphetamines, methylphenidate (Ritalin), barbiturates, pholcodine.
Class C: the least harmful	Tranquillisers, some painkillers, GHB (gammahydroxybutyrate), ketamine, anabolic steroids, benzodiazepines, growth hormones.

Table 2.1: Classification of drugs under the Misuse of Drugs Act 1971

and can be moved between classes. The full list is extensive, but any nurse would be expected to know about the range of these drugs that can be prescribed for use in healthcare. It is important for all healthcare professionals to comply with the law at all times, and the management of CD usage has been much more tightly controlled since the Shipman Enquiry reports (2002–5).

The Misuse of Drugs Regulations 2001 defines who is allowed to supply and possess CDs while acting in a health professional capacity, and lays down the conditions under which these activities may legitimately be carried out (HMSO, 1973/2001). There are five schedules under the regulations, each of which details the requirements for import, export, production, supply, possession, prescription and record keeping of specific drugs named in the five schedules (see Table 2.2). As a student you do not need to know this in detail, but you would nevertheless be expected to know about a variety of CDs in common use in healthcare.

Use of controlled drugs in healthcare

While many of the drugs identified in the Misuse of Drugs Act 1971 have no recognised therapeutic use, there are others that are very useful in the care and treatment of patients with terminal disease for the relief of pain, for the relief of post-operative pain, for the relief of severe acute pain (for example, a fractured bone) and for anaesthesia. For example, morphine is commonly used for severe pain. These drugs are often prescribed to patients in hospital and in their own homes, and the Misuse of Drugs Regulations 2001 are there to ensure these drugs are managed properly and within the law (HMSO, 1973/2001). Such controls will be included in a written medicines management policy in a hospital or other clinical area and all staff will be expected to maintain compliance with this policy at all times. Transgressions of such policies will be taken very seriously by employers. Nursing students are also expected to comply with such policies, and will also be required to comply with any policy set by their university. All healthcare professionals must also comply with Standard Operating Procedures, as described below.

Schedule	Examples of drugs in each schedule
Schedule 1	Cannabis and cannabinoids.
Schedule 2	Opiate-based drugs used in acute palliative care.
Schedule 3	Substances less likely to be open to abuse than those in Schedule 2, such as synthetic opioids and some powerful herbal medicines.
Schedule 4	Prescription-only medicines (Part 1 – benzodiazepines and zolpidam; Part 2 – anabolic steroids).
Schedule 5	Medicines that contain very low dosages of drugs, such as codeine and pholcodeine.

Table 2.2: Schedules of drugs under the Misuse of Drugs Regulations 2001

Standard Operating Procedures in relation to controlled drugs

The Health Act 2006 requires each healthcare organisation (e.g. hospital Trust, Primary Care Trust (PCT), hospice) to appoint an Accountable Officer, responsible for the safe and effective use of controlled drugs and to introduce Standard Operating Procedures (SOPs) for the use and management of CDs. In addition, GP practices need to have processes in place to agree and adopt SOPs for their use.

Guidance from the Department of Health states that a Standard Operating Procedure is a document that describes the responsibilities and the procedures, including audit, necessary to manage CDs safely and accountably. The guidance is explicit in what the SOP should include:

- ordering and receipt of CDs;
- assigning responsibilities;
- storage of CDs;
- persons who can have access to the CDs;
- security in storage and transportation of CDs as required by Misuse of Drugs legislation;
- disposal and destruction of CDs;
- who is to be alerted if complications arise;
- record keeping, including:
  - maintaining relevant CD registers under Misuse of Drugs legislation;
  - maintaining a record of the CDs specified in Schedule 2 to the Misuse of Drugs Regulations 2001 that have been returned by patients.

The GP practice SOP should also include:

- responsibilities within the practice team;
- validation by the PCT organisation and date;
- review period, e.g. one, two or three years;
- lead author and named people contributing to the SOP.

The following activity is designed to help you become familiar with the management of CDs in the clinical area where you undertake your placement, and with finding information from the BNF. We will then go on to discuss in more detail the ordering, delivery, storage and labelling of CDs.

Activity 2.2　　　　　　　　　　　　　　　　　　　*Critical thinking*

Think about the way controlled drugs were handled during your most recent practice learning opportunity.

1. Where was the CD storage cupboard located? Think about the position of this cupboard and the information you have read in this chapter; do you think that it is positioned appropriately and why?
2. Where were the CD record and requisition books located? Why is it important that storage of these items is in a secure place?

continued overleaf . . .

continued . . .

3. Select one of the CDs listed in the record book (for example, morphine sulphate) and locate the entry relating to it in the BNF. Then answer the following questions.
    (a) What preparations and dosages of the medicine are available?
    (b) How should the medicine be administered?
    (c) What are the expected therapeutic effects of this medicine?
    (d) How would you monitor that these therapeutic effects occur?
    (e) What side effects could occur as the result of taking this medicine?
    (f) How would you monitor for the occurrence of side effects?

An outline answer is provided at the end of the chapter.

Ordering and delivery of CDs to wards and departments in hospitals

When you are working in a hospital, these are the procedures you will follow.

CDs required for wards and departments must be ordered from the pharmacy by the Sister or acting Sister. (This was the term in common use when the legislation was enacted; it would be now interpreted as the nurse in charge of the ward, and the deputy.) CDs must be ordered in a book specifically for that purpose.

The following information should be given in the order:

- name of the CD in BLOCK LETTERS;
- the formulation required (e.g. tablets, ampoules for injection);
- the strength required in both words and figures;
- the total quantity required.

Each preparation requested should be written on a separate page of the order book. The requisition should be signed and dated, and the nurse ordering the CD should add his or her job designation to the order. The whole order book is sent to the pharmacy, where the requisition is made up by the pharmacist who then signs the order.

The order must be delivered in a safe and secure manner to the ward or department by the person who must also sign as the 'messenger'.

The pages in the requisition books are numbered and in duplicate. The top page is retained by the pharmacy and the duplicate (pink) page stays in the book.

CDs may be delivered to wards in locked boxes or by a designated person considered suitable for that purpose. This could be a nursing student, but consideration needs to be taken of whether or not being a pharmacy messenger is a suitable role for a student other than in the context of learning about the management of CDs.

When the CD and order book are returned to the ward, the CDs need to be checked and taken on to the ward stock. A registered nurse and one other person should check that the CD supplied is in accordance with the requisition. The other person can be a student nurse acting under supervision of the registered nurse, so long as he or she understands the principles of accurate record keeping. The order book is then signed to indicate that the CD has been received. If there are any problems identified, the pharmacy should be notified immediately.

Each ward should have a **controlled drugs record book** in which all CDs received on the ward and given to patients are recorded. An entry of the new supply is made in the record book.

Each CD and each different form, strength and preparation of a CD should have a separate page in the record book. An index to pages should be in the front of the book and amended as required.

New stock of a CD can be added to existing stock on the appropriate page. This stock must be properly stored and labelled, as described in the next two sections.

Storage of controlled drugs

Because CDs are those that are liable to abuse and misuse, they must be safely and securely stored on the ward, and access to them must be strictly controlled.

CDs must be stored in a separate locked cupboard to which unauthorised access is prevented. Often this cupboard is contained within another medicines cupboard. The CD cupboard should not be used for any other purpose. It may have a light to indicate when it is open.

The cupboard should be in a visible place so that it can be seen by nurses working on the ward. However, it is best to avoid very busy places, as the nurses preparing and checking CDs must be able to concentrate on the task in hand.

The keys to the cupboard should be kept safely on the person of the nurse in charge of the ward, and must be separate from other keys in use. Spare keys should be kept in the pharmacy or, if there is no pharmacy, in a safe place in the hospital. In departments where there is not 24-hour staffing, keys must be kept securely when the department is not staffed.

Lost or missing keys should be reported to the senior nurse on duty, who will inform the pharmacy.

Activity 2.3   *Decision-making*

You are on duty, observing the dispensing of a CD from the CD cupboard by two staff nurses. They notice that there is a discrepancy between the stock amount of the CD as recorded in the CD record book and the number of tablets actually in the packaging. The CD record book records that there should be 15 tablets in stock, but the actual tablet count is only 14.

*   What actions would you expect the staff nurses to take on discovering this discrepancy?

An outline answer is provided at the end of the chapter.

Labelling of medicines

All medicines, whether bought over the counter or provided on prescription, must be clearly labelled. The 1968 Act describes what labelling is required (HMSO, 1968). The label should be written in English and be legible, clear and comprehensible. When giving medicines to patients in hospital or in their own homes, the nurse should be satisfied that the information on the label is clear. If in doubt, the medicine should not be given until advice is sought. Patients should be actively discouraged from removing medicines from the original container. The information on an original manufacturer's container must include the following:

- the product name – preferably the approved name, but a **proprietary** or **trade name** may also be used;
- the form the medicine is to take (the pharmaceutical form), such as tablets or capsules;
- the route or method of administration;
- the product strength, giving both **active** and **non-active ingredients** (**excipients**); for some medicines (injectable, eye and topical preparations), all non-active ingredients must be stated;
- the amount of the medicine in the container, for example the number of tablets (dosage units) or weight of a cream or ointment or the amount in millilitres (mls) in a suspension of eye drops;
- any excipient known to have a recognised action;
- special storage instructions – for example, storage in a cool place;
- the expiry date, after which the medicine should not be used – usually given as the month and year;
- name and address of the holder of the authorisation to market the medicine and the authorisation number;
- the reference number of the batch;
- instructions for use;
- any special instructions for disposal.

When a medicine is dispensed by a pharmacist as a prescription, extra labelling is required. Manufacturers' containers may have a space where this label can be placed. Additional information can be contained on the patient information leaflet, which should be in each medicines container. Further information about patient information leaflets is given later in this chapter.

In addition to Standard Operating Procedures just described, there is a great deal of professional guidance available of which nurses should be aware.

Professional guidance on the management of medicines

Hospital policies on medicines management

All hospitals will have a written policy on medicines management, and all staff will be required to be familiar with its contents and comply with its requirements. Hospital policies are set out within the context of current legal and professional requirements and should take into account the following.

- The Medicines Act 1968 and subsequent amendments (HMSO, 1968).
- The Misuse of Drugs Act 1971 and subsequent amendments (HMSO, 1971).
- The Misuse of Drugs Regulations 1973 and 2001 and subsequent amendments (HMSO, 1973/2001).
- The Aitken Report, 1958 – *Control of Dangerous Drugs and Poisons within Hospitals.* This report followed a government initiated inquiry into how dangerous drugs and poisons were controlled in hospitals and indicated that pharmacists were the professionals who were responsible for medicines in the hospital as a whole and not just responsible for them in the pharmacy. This led to the safer administration of medicines and the introduction of standard prescription sheets for individual patients. Pharmacists then became much more involved with medicines at ward level (Anderson, 2005, pp241–3).
- The Roxburgh Report, 1972 – *Control of Medicines in Hospital Wards and Departments* (Anderson, 2005, pp241–3).
- The Duthie Report, 1988 – *Guidelines for the Safe and Secure Handling of Medicines* (Anderson, 2005, pp241–3).
- Controlled Drugs (Supervision of Management and Use) Regulations 2006 (HMSO, 2006).
- Department of Health guidance – *Safer Management of Controlled Drugs* (DH, 2006).
- Department of Health guidance – *Safer Management of Controlled Drugs: Early action* (DH, 2007a).
- *The Code: Standards of conduct, performance and ethics for nurses and midwives* (NMC, 2008).
- *Standards for Medicines Management* (NMC, 2007b).
- *Record Keeping: Guidance for nurses and midwives* (NMC, 2009).

A hospital or Trust policy for medicines management may contain a number of sections addressing various aspects of medicines management, or there may be a number of different policies addressing different aspects. For example, a policy on the administration of CDs should contain information about legislation and the responsibilities of staff – who is entitled to check and administer CDs and a detailed section on the procedure for administration. A policy should also contain a statement about what nursing students are allowed to do in relation to medicines management. For example, it would be possible for a nursing student to be allowed to act as a second checker for CDs once they have undertaken relevant instruction within their university. It is important for you as a student to ask to see any medicines management policy at the start of your first clinical placement in a hospital or other clinical area. This may be available on a local intranet.

University policies for students

Your university should provide you with access to its own medicines management policy, which you must follow at all times. This policy is likely to detail what you are allowed to undertake as a student, and also what you are not allowed to do. Policies may differ between fields of practice and will take into account the requirements of the university's partner Trusts where placements are provided. The university should make its policy available to Trusts where its students undertake practice placements, so that Trusts are aware of the university's expectations of its students. Any policy should adhere to current NMC and legal requirements.

A university medicines management policy for nursing students should show:

- which students the guidance is intended for (adult, child, mental health or learning disability student nurses);
- how the university policy links with medicines management policies of partner Trusts; the university policy should be decided in consultation with nursing representation from hospital Trusts that provide the placements for students;
- how students should use opportunities to participate in medicines management while on placements;
- the criteria that a student must have met in order to be allowed to participate in medicines management; for example, he or she should have attended the university taught sessions on medicines management;
- which aspects of medicines management students are allowed to participate in; for example, a student can administer oral medication to a patient if he or she has acted as a checker, and is doing so under the direct supervision of a registered nurse;
- which aspects of medicines management students are not allowed to participate in; for example, while a student may observe the administration of intravenous medication, he or she would not be permitted to administer it as it is currently a skill that does not fall within pre-registration training.

Activity 2.4 — *Evidence-based practice*

- Locate and familiarise yourself with your university's medicines management policy for nursing students. You may have been provided with a copy of this when you started the course; alternatively, it may be available on your university's intranet site, such as Blackboard.
- When you are next on clinical placement, ask your mentor to show you the medicines management policy for your hospital Trust. Does it contain any specific information detailing the roles and responsibilities of the nursing student in medicines management?

As this is an individual activity there is no outline answer provided.

The Nursing and Midwifery Council

The Nursing and Midwifery Council (NMC), which *exists to safeguard the health and wellbeing of the public*, publishes guidance and standards for registered practitioners to help them discharge their responsibilities as nurses. The NMC is also responsible for setting the standards for the training of nurses in the UK and in this respect students are expected to be compliant with *The Code: Standards of conduct, performance and ethics for nurses and midwives* (2008), and with the *Standards for Medicines Management* (2007b).

NMC *Standards for Medicines Management* 2007

Standards 18 and 19 apply specifically to nursing students.

- Standard 18 states: *Students must never administer/supply medicinal products without direct supervision.*
- Standard 19 states: *In delegating the administration of medicinal products to unregistered practitioners, it is the registrant who must apply the principles of administration of medicinal products as listed above. They may then delegate an unregistered practitioner to assist the patient in the ingestion or application of the medicinal product.*

The role of the student in these respects is clear. As a student you cannot administer a medical product to a patient unless you are directly supervised by a registered nurse, and if you are asked to do so unsupervised, you must refuse. These publications are available in paper format and online, and they are reviewed on a regular basis. You should make yourself familiar with these publications, as it is important that you know the guidance the NMC gives to its registrants. The *Standards for Medicines Management* includes a CD-ROM, about which the NMC states *it is essential to read the full guidance and you must follow the advice.* The guidance and standards are in all respects compliant with the law.

As well as complying with SOPs and being aware of the professional guidance available, nurses must adhere to a code of ethics when dealing with the administration and management of medicines. These will now be discussed, with special emphasis on consent and on covert administration.

Ethics and medicines management

Patients have the personal choice whether or not to take medicines that are prescribed for them. Having offered themselves for assessment, diagnosis and treatment, most people would choose to take the medicines that are prescribed for them. However, *The Code* (2008, p4) makes it clear that *you must ensure that you gain consent before you begin any treatment or care.* Normally, it would not be necessary to obtain written consent, or to ask a direct question to obtain consent when administering medication. This is because consent to the administration of medicines can be implied when, for example, the patient holds out their hand to receive tablets, or bares a limb for an injection. However, a patient may refuse to take prescribed medication, and this raises a number of ethical issues. The law assumes that a person of adult years has the mental capacity to give or refuse consent to treatment. The Mental Capacity Act 2005 empowers and protects people who are not able to make their own decisions and defines mental capacity as *having the ability to comprehend and retain treatment information, being able to believe the information given, being able to weigh up the pros and cons of the information and being able to communicate a decision* (HMSO, 2005). The test of mental capacity asks if a person has an impairment of mind or brain, or a disturbance of mental function; in other words, are they able to make the decision in question at the time it needs to be made? The NMC *Code* (2008, p4) states that *you must respect and support people's rights to accept or decline treatment or care.* Taken in the context of medicines administration, this means that, if a patient declines medication, you cannot take it upon yourself to insist to the patient that they must take the medicine. Clearly, there are some instances where obtaining consent is problematical, such as in emergency situations where the immediate administration of medicines or other treatment and care could be a life-saving measure.

Consent by children to the administration of medicines

The law assumes that children under the age of 16 years lack the necessary mental capacity to consent or not to treatment and care, which includes the administration of medicines, and it is parents who have the right to make health-related decisions for their children. However, some children under the age of 16, if they show significant understanding and intelligence, can be allowed to decide for themselves about whether or not to take medication, or to give or refuse their own consent to care and treatment (NSPCC, 1985). Refusal of consent by a child up to the age of 18 can be overridden by parents in England and Wales, but not in Scotland. Only very rarely is the intervention of the courts required to establish what is right for the child in cases of differing views.

The following activity will help you to assist in making decisions in unexpected situations.

Activity 2.5   *Evidence-based practice*

You are on a practice learning opportunity in a children's ward. You are assisting a registered nurse to administer an antibiotic to a two-year-old child. The child swallows about half the dose, but spits out the rest.

1. How should this be recorded?
2. Should you give the child some more antibiotic to make up for what has been spat out?
3. What other actions could you and the registered nurse take?

An outline answer is provided at the end of the chapter.

Consent by mental health clients to the administration of medicines

In some situations in a mental healthcare and treatment context, a decision may be made under the Mental Health Act 2007 (HMSO, 2007) that medicines treatment can be given without the patient's consent. This would be to either save the patient's life, or reduce serious suffering, or prevent the patient's condition from becoming worse or prevent violent behaviour or danger to the patient or others. This treatment cannot carry on indefinitely and, after three months of treatment with medication, the doctor must obtain the consent of the patient for it to carry on. If such consent is not forthcoming, there are clear steps that need to be taken that involve an independent second opinion by a doctor, who will discuss the proposed treatment with the patient and staff caring for him or her.

Covert administration of medicines

The notion of informed consent with regard to medicines administration implies that patients have adequate information about the nature, purpose and effects of the medicines that are prescribed; that their consent to receive medicines is freely given and not obtained under pressure, duress or coercion; and finally that the patient has the capacity to consent – they understand everything about the purpose of the medication, the risks and benefits of taking it and the consequences of choosing not to take it. The issue of consent is important because many nurses and doctors would feel that it is always in a patient's best interests for them to take the medication prescribed and would perhaps seek ways to ensure that this happens as they see the administration of medicines as a beneficial act. However, it is not generally acceptable to disguise medication so that it is given covertly to patients. The NMC (2007a) defines covert administration as *disguising medicine in food or drink, so that a patient or client is led to believe that they are not receiving medicine, when in fact they are.* Anecdotal evidence exists that covert administration does takes place, and that it is relatively common.

In 2007 the NMC issued advice on the covert administration of medicines. This is currently in the process of being updated, but these general points describe the current position.

- *The covert administration of medicines is only likely to be necessary or appropriate in the case of patients or clients who actively refuse medication but who are judged not to have the capacity to understand the consequences of their refusal.*
- *The NMC recognises that there may be certain exceptional circumstances in which covert administration may be considered to prevent a patient/client from missing out on essential treatment. In such circumstances and in the absence of informed consent, the following considerations may apply:*
  - *The best interests of the patient/client must be considered at all times.*
  - *The medication must be considered essential for the patient's/client's health and well-being, or for the safety of others.*
  - *The decision to administer a medication covertly should not be considered routine, and should be a contingency measure. Any decision to do so must be reached after assessing the care needs of the patient/client individually. It should be patient/client-specific, in order to avoid the ritualised administration of medication in this way.*
  - *There should be broad and open discussion among the multi-professional clinical team and the supporters of the patient/client, and agreement that this approach is required in the circumstances. Those involved should include carers, relatives, advocates, and the multidisciplinary team (especially the pharmacist). Family involvement in the care process should be positively encouraged. The method of administration of the medicines should be agreed with the pharmacist.*
  - *The decision and the action taken, including the names of all parties concerned, should be documented in the care plan and reviewed at appropriate intervals.*
  - *Regular attempts should be made to encourage the patient/client to take their medication. This might best be achieved by giving regular information, explanation and encouragement, preferably by the team member who has the best rapport with the individual.*

(NMC, 2007a)

Therefore, Trusts and other healthcare provider organisations should take these nursing professional practice guidelines into consideration when medicines management policy is formulated.

As nurses, unless there is clear evidence to the contrary, we should always assume that the patients we look after have the mental capacity to make decisions about their own care. We should always ensure that we have obtained consent from patients to give them their prescribed medication. If a patient declines medication, a record should be kept, both on the medicines administration chart and in any nursing notes. The patient's doctor should be informed. Because nurses should always be acting in the best interests of their patients, they should make sure that they always continue to encourage patients to take their prescribed medication. Nurses should seek out ways of making medicines more palatable for patients, as sometimes refusal is because medicines may be difficult to take – they may smell or taste unpleasant, or have side effects that patients do not want to tolerate. Elderly clients or children may find swallowing pills or tablets difficult and a liquid formation may well be more acceptable. Discussion with the patient's doctors and the pharmacist is essential. As a student you should always inform your mentor or other nurse working in your placement area if your patient declines or refuses medicines that you administer. Try to be involved in discussions about how to resolve situations in the patient's best interests.

The following activity is designed to help you think about ethical issues related to medicines management. The chapter will then conclude by examining the various sources of information about medicines that nurses can consult.

Activity 2.6   *Decision-making*

You are attending a placement on a ward caring for older people. You notice that one of the patients consistently spits out capsules, and has considerable difficulty swallowing all her medicines, even with lots of encouragement from the nurses and copious amounts of water.

The patient's relatives state that, at home, they normally crush all the medication and empty the capsules into spoonfuls of jam or sugar to make sure that it is swallowed, and they suggest that the same is done in hospital.

1. How should the nursing staff respond to this suggestion?
2. What measures could be taken to ensure that the patient receives her medication?

An outline answer is provided at the end of the chapter.

Where to find out about medicines

When a nurse administers a medicine to a patient, it is essential that he or she knows about that medicine. The NMC *Standards for Medicines Management* states the following:

> *the administration of medicines is an important aspect of the professional practice of persons whose names are on the Council's register. It is not solely a mechanistic task to be performed in strict compliance with the written prescription of a medical practitioner (now independent/supplementary prescriber). It requires thought and the exercise of professional judgement.*

(2007b, p1)

Professional judgement thus implies that, each time a nurse administers a medicine to a patient, knowledge of that medicine is essential. For each medicine given to a patient the nurse should know the normal dosage, the expected effect and how to monitor for that effect, what side effects may occur and how to recognise these, and any interactions with other medicines. In the course of giving medicines to patients, for example in the context of a 'medicines round', the nurse should be able to consult that information quickly, so that an informed judgement can be made about whether or not administering the medicine is an appropriate professional action. Experienced registered nurses will have accumulated a large amount of knowledge about the medicines that are prescribed and administered in their own area of practice. However, as a nursing student you will not yet have that knowledge and experience, so you must know what sources are available to you to find out about medicines. Not only do you need to know this for yourself, so that you are safe and competent to act as the assistant to a registered nurse administering medicines, but you also need to know so that you can educate your patients and carers in the future about medicines.

The *British National Formulary*

The *British National Formulary* (BNF) is by far the most popular source for medicines knowledge. As well as being intended for medical practitioners and pharmacists, it is also for use by other healthcare professionals and aims to provide them with sound up-to-date information about the use of medicines. It is used extensively by nurses undertaking medicines administration as it provides a rapid method of obtaining the basic information required for safe administration. The BNF is a joint publication of the BMJ (British Medical Journal) Publishing Group and the Royal Pharmaceutical Society of Great Britain. Published twice a year, each edition is numbered and dated, and it is important that a recent edition is available on a ward or in another clinical area for nurses to consult during the administration of medicines. A prescriber should always use the most recent edition. The BNF is also available online and as an application ('app') for a mobile phone. This would be useful for community prescribers who are in patients' homes when prescribing decisions may need to be made.

Other publications in the BNF series are the *British National Formulary for Children* (BNFC, 2009), and the *Nurse Prescribers' Formulary for Community Practitioners* (NPF, 2009–11). The children's formulary should be available for consultation when working in any area where children are nursed, and if you accompany a community nurse who is a prescriber, the NPF should be available for consultation.

Medicines information sheets

When you buy a GSL or P medicines, or when a patient is prescribed a prescription-only medicine (POM) in the community, each package of medication should contain a patient information leaflet. These leaflets provide comprehensive information to patients about the medicines they are taking, including what the medicine is used for, what to do and know before the medicine is taken, how to take the medicine, possible side effects, how to store the medicine and any further information that the manufacturer considers necessary. Patients in hospital who are given their medicines by nurses during the course of their hospital stay do not have these information sheets to look at, so the nurse must be prepared to answer a patient's questions about their medicines in such a way that the information is accurate, yet easy to understand. The BNF will not provide these kinds of details, so as a student you should look at the information sheets and use this kind of knowledge when required. When a patient is discharged from hospital with take-home medication, the information leaflets should be provided for them. An online site is available for access to many of these patient information leaflets, and some are also available in accessible formats on request, for example in large print or Braille format for sight-impaired people.

Online information

As well as the BNF online, there are a number of other online sources for medicines knowledge. When you type the name of a medicine into an internet search engine, there may be tens of thousands of results. It is important therefore that any site you choose to look at must be a reliable and authoritative site. You also need to make sure that any website you choose to consult is a UK site. Medicine names and legislation still differ from country to country, and you need UK-specific knowledge to administer medicines safely in UK healthcare institutions, especially with regard to legislation.

The National Institute for Health and Clinical Excellence

The National Institute for Health and Clinical Excellence (NICE) was set up in 2004 in the government White Paper, *Choosing Health: Making healthier choices*. Its role is to *bring together knowledge and guidance on ways of promoting good health and treating ill health*. Thus, part of its role is the evaluation of medicines new to the market, as well as existing medicines, as part of clinical guidelines that NHS staff must follow in the management of disease. NICE has been criticised for taking too long to recommend and produce guidance, particularly in relation to new anti-cancer drugs. However, each set of clinical guidelines has been produced only after extensive research by an appointed group of people, including health professional staff, and lay and patient repre-sentatives, and incorporates evidence-based best clinical practice as well as drug treatment guidance. Nurses can be reassured, therefore, that the medicines they administer to patients for specific conditions are the best and most cost-effective method of treatment for that condition. NHS professionals are expected to implement NICE recommendations within three months of publication.

Medicines safety

It is important that the medicines that people can buy and those that are prescribed by an authorised health professional for treatment of an illness or other purpose are safe to take. Many medicines have side effects, but this does not preclude them from being prescribed; however, it makes sense that medicines should do good rather than harm. Over the years, many intrinsically dangerous substances have been given to people as medicine for the treatment of disease. For example, at one time mercury was a treatment for syphilis – a sexually transmitted disease. Dangerous poisons such as arsenic have also been used in the past. As the detrimental effects of these substances were recognised and better, more effective treatments emerged, so they were withdrawn from use (Anderson, 2005, pp244–5). As health professionals we can be sure that the medicines we administer to our patients have been through clinical trials to establish their safety and effectiveness long before they become available for human clinical use. This is the responsibility of the Commission on Human Medicines (CHM), which is part of the Medicines and Healthcare products Regulatory Agency (MHRA) – the government agency that is responsible for determining the safety of medicines and a wide range of other healthcare products. It carries out its role in a number of ways, and ensures that the safety and quality standards of all healthcare products comply with European and UK laws and regulations.

The CHM/MHRA operate the 'Yellow Card' system, by which health professionals can report suspected adverse drug reactions. An example of a 'Yellow Card' can be found in the back of the BNF. The MHRA keeps a register of these suspected side effects, and this helps to provide early warnings of potential drug hazards. The MHRA also issues a monthly Drug Safety update, which contains the latest advice on aspects of drug safety that health professionals need to know. Doctors and pharmacists are encouraged to register to receive the update online. Another of the MHRA's roles is to assess misleading or incorrect information contained in advertisements for medicines, product labels and product information leaflets. Thus, the public and the health professions can be reassured that the information given to them is as accurate as possible.

NICE and the MHRA have differing but complementary roles. The MHRA decides if a medicine is safe and can be made available for sale, whereas the role of NICE is to establish whether a medicine is appropriate for use in a particular clinical context and to recommend its use.

Chapter summary

This chapter has introduced the professional, legal and ethical context of medicines management that you as a student nurse in the first year of your training programme should be expected to know. The NMC expects you to have this information to hand, in order to act in a safe and competent way when assisting registered nurses in their role of administering medicines to patients. Medicines legislation and regulation is complex. The Medicines Act 1968 is the legal basis by which medicines are tested, manufactured, licensed and sold (HMSO, 1968). The Medicines and Health Products Regulatory Agency, including the Commission on Human Medicines, is the body through which the law is enacted and interpreted for manufacturers, doctors, pharmacists and nurses. The National Institute for Clinical Excellence decides which medicines will be made available to patients for their treatment. You can find out about these medicines by consulting one of the sources mentioned in the chapter.

Activities: brief outline answers

Activity 2.1 Categories of medicine (page 49)

GSL	P	POM
Ibuprofen	Piriton	Codeine phosphate
Paracetamol	Ranitidine	Salbutamol
Bonjela	Chloramphenicol eye drops	Bacillus Calmette-Guerin (BCG) vaccine

Activity 2.2 Handling, storage and management of controlled drugs (pages 51–2)

1. The guidance in the chapter states that the CD cupboard should be located in an area where it can be seen, but in such a place that nurses are not disturbed or interrupted while they are preparing CDs. The location will depend on the ward design; in modern hospitals, they can often be found sited at the nurses' station. In older hospitals they may be found in treatment rooms, or at one end of the ward near the ward office.
2. The CD record book should be kept near the cupboard, so that it is immediately accessible when a CD is prepared. It should be taken to the patient's bedside when the CD is administered and returned to its normal place afterwards.

    The CD requisition book should be kept securely in an appropriate place, for example locked in the ward office. This is to ensure that it is not lost or stolen.
3. The answer given is for morphine:

    The *British National Formulary* contains a large amount of information about opioid analgesics (pain killers) of which morphine is one example. Make sure that you read all the general information about opioid medicines as well as the specific information about morphine. Opioid analgesics are medicines that have their main action on the central nervous system and are controlled drugs because of their addictive qualities. The information given below is a summary and does not replace a full reading of the relevant section in the BNF. You may find it helpful to summarise information about other medicines in the same way, so that you become familiar with using the BNF as well as learning about medicines. The NMC *Standards for Medicines Management*, standard 8, states that *you must know the therapeutic uses of the medicine to be administered, its normal dosage, side effects, precautions and contra-indications.*

*   Preparations available: oral solutions, tablets, modified release tablets, suppositories, injections, injections with an anti-emetic.

    The dosage range depends upon the age of the patient and the reason for administration and needs to be adjusted for each individual patient. Post-operative pain in a normal adult may require 5–10mg every four hours. It is important that the dose is adjusted by the prescriber according to the effect and side effects.
*   Methods of administration: oral solutions, tablets and sustained release tablets by mouth, suppositories per rectum; injections by the intramuscular, subcutaneous and intravenous routes.
*   Expected therapeutic effects: morphine is given for moderate to severe pain, particularly of visceral origin (pain arising from internal body organs). It can be used in acute pain situations, and is also used for the treatment of pain in palliative care. The expected therapeutic effect is that of pain relief; however, **dependence** and **tolerance** may occur over time where a larger dose is required to achieve the same analgesic effect.
*   Monitoring for expected effectiveness: the patient should be closely monitored to check that pain has been relieved; a recognised pain chart or scale can be helpful to both nurse and patient in monitoring the analgesic effect.
*   Side effects that may occur: the most common side effects are nausea and vomiting, constipation and a dry mouth; larger doses may cause respiratory depression, hypotension and a wide range of central nervous system effects.
*   Monitoring for side effects: the patient should be asked to report any effect that causes discomfort, especially nausea and vomiting where an anti-emetic (anti-sickness) drug can be prescribed. The patient's respiratory rate and effort and blood pressure should be recorded regularly. Other side effects such as drowsiness will be readily apparent.

Activity 2.3 Dealing with discrepancies (page 53)

*   The staff nurses should recount the stock dosage, just in case they initially miscounted. They should check back in the CD record book to ensure that totals have been added/deducted correctly.
*   It would be advisable to check the CD cupboard for any tablets that may have fallen out of their packaging.

- The staff nurses could check patients' medicine charts to ascertain those patients that have been administered the CD since the last stock check, checking also that the dose administered is the dose recorded in the CD record book.
- The pharmacist should be contacted and asked to check the total amount of the CD they last sent to the ward.
- If all these checks fail to reveal where the discrepancy originated, this incident must be reported to the ward manager and pharmacist and an incident form should be completed in line with Trust policy.

Activity 2.5 Child's rejection of medicine (page 58)

1. The registered nurse should record in the appropriate place on the medicine chart that the child received only some of the antibiotic and refused the rest. This information should also be written in any nursing notes. Standard 8 of the NMC *Standards for Medicines Management* states that *you must make a clear, accurate and immediate record of all medicine administered, intentionally withheld or refused by the patient, ensuring that the signature is clear and legible.*
2. It is not advisable to give another dose, as it could not be certain how much the child has taken.
3. The doctor should be informed, and alternative ways of administering the antibiotic should be discussed. Parents or carers could become involved in helping the child to take the medicine if considered appropriate.

Activity 2.6 Covert administration of medicines (page 60)

1. If you refer back to the section on covert administration of medicines (pp59–60), it is clear that this suggestion could only be acted on if the patient consents to the medicines being given in this way, assuming that the patient has the mental capacity to do so. The nursing staff should check the hospital medicines management policy to see if there is any agreed protocol in place to deal with such a situation. There should be discussion with the patient and with all those involved with the patient's care, including the relatives, and a decision should be made.
2. Elderly patients often find it difficult to swallow medicines in tablet or capsule form. This can be for a number of reasons, such as the size and shape of the medicine, an unpleasant taste, ill-fitting false teeth, or a dry mouth and throat. Many medicines are available in preparations other than capsules or tablets, so discussion with the doctor and pharmacist could result in the medicines being prescribed in a liquid format that is easier to swallow. It is important not to rush when helping elderly patients to swallow medicines. Being patient and taking time may be all that is needed. The patient may be entirely happy to have his or her medicines crushed up in jam or sugar, but the nursing staff must check with the pharmacist to ensure that this is appropriate for each of the medicines.

Knowledge review

Now that you've worked through the chapter, how would you rate your knowledge of the following topics?

	Good	Adequate	Poor
1. The legal and regulatory frameworks in which medicines management takes place.			
2. Medicines management in a professional and ethical context.			
3. How to find up-to-date information about all kinds of medicines.			

Where you're not confident in your knowledge of a topic, what will you do next?

Further reading

Dimond, B (2005) *Legal Aspects of Medicines*. London: Quay Books.

This book offers useful information on the law and legislation governing various aspects of medicines management.

Hendrick, J (2010). *Law and Ethics in Children's Nursing*. Chichester: Wiley-Blackwell.

This book offers an introduction to law and ethics in children; it deals with the principles of autonomy and consent in children.

Jevon, P, Payne, E, Higgins, D and Endacott, R (2010) *Medicines Management: A guide for nurses.* Chichester: Wiley-Blackwell.

Chapter 2 of this book provides information on the various legal aspects of medicines management.

Useful websites

www.legislation.gov.uk

This website publishes a variety of legislation related to many different aspects of the law, including medicines management.

www.medicinesforchildren.org.uk/index.php

This website provides information leaflets about the use of medicines in children. They are written for parents and carers but will also be suitable for older children.

www.mhra.gov.uk

This website provides useful information on the role of the Medicines and Healthcare products Regulatory Agency in ensuring that medicines and medical products are safe to use.

www.mhra.gov.uk/Committees/Medicinesadvisorybodies/CommissiononHumanMedicines/index.htm

This is the website of the Commission on Human Medicines.

www.nice.org.uk

This is the website of the National Institute for Health and Clinical Excellence.

www.npc.co.uk/mm/publications.htm

This is a useful website from the NHS National Prescribing Centre that provides a variety of publications related to medicines management.

www.patient.co.uk/dils.asp

Medicines information sheets for patients are available here.

www.the-shipman-inquiry.org.uk

This website sets out in detail the circumstances and subsequent inquiry that enabled a general practitioner to murder patients in his care by misusing medicines.

Chapter 3
The principles of pharmacology

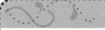
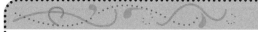

continued . . . .

Cluster: Medicines management

36. People can trust the newly registered graduate nurse to ensure safe and effective practice in medicines management through comprehensive knowledge of medicines, their actions, risks and benefits.

By the second progression point:

1. Uses knowledge of commonly administered medicines in order to act promptly in cases where side effects and adverse reactions occur.

Chapter aims

By the end of this chapter, you should be able to:

* understand the principles of pharmacodynamics and pharmacokinetics;
* discuss factors affecting the pharmacodynamics and pharmacokinetics of medicines.

Introduction

Case study

Mary Santini is a 70-year-old lady. She was admitted to the Accident and Emergency Department after being found on the floor at home by her neighbour. She has sustained a fracture to the neck of her left femur and bruising to her temple. Mary's neighbour has brought her medication into the department. She is taking lithium for her bipolar disorder. Mary is in pain, but since she has bruising to her temple, the doctors need to rule out a possible head injury. They are reluctant to prescribe her morphine, due to its sedative properties, which may mask any signs or symptoms of a head injury, and have decided to prescribe diclofenac instead. Two weeks later Mary has recovered from the surgery to her fractured neck of femur. She is well enough to go home and has been discharged with a supply of her lithium medicine and diclofenac for pain relief. Three weeks later Mary dies.

Had the doctors and nurses understood that patients receiving lithium can accumulate toxic levels of lithium in the bloodstream when taking diclofenac, they would not have prescribed or administered diclofenac in this case. Mary might still be alive. While this is a fictitious scenario, such cases do too often occur, and they could so easily be avoided if doctors and nurses understood the basic principles of pharmacology and medicine interactions.

This chapter will enable you to understand how medicines work in the body (**pharmaco-dynamics**) and how medicines are **absorbed**, **distributed**, **metabolised** and **excreted** (**pharmacokinetics**) from the body. It is important that you learn the principles of pharmacokinetics and pharmacodynamics to enable you to understand how medicines work and therefore be aware of any possible **adverse reactions** to medicines. This will enable you to take appropriate action should your patient suffer any such effects. It is also necessary to understand the various factors that affect the pharmacodynamics and pharmacokinetics of medicines for your particular patient group, for example the route of administration and the age, sex, nutritional status, illness, body weight, genetics and ethnicity of the patient.

You may feel quite daunted when it comes to trying to understand pharmacological principles and how they apply to specific medicines and relate to your nursing practice. It is neither necessary nor possible to know the name and function of every single medicine that is available. You should concentrate on becoming familiar with the processes involved in the **pharmacology** of medicines and then be able to apply them to common groups of medicines that you will encounter in your nursing practice.

As a foundation-year student the NMC (2010a, b) requires you to ensure that your practice is safe and effective. You can demonstrate this through comprehensive knowledge of medicines and their actions, risks and benefits. In order to pass through the second progression point in your programme you must be able to prove that you have acquired the necessary knowledge of commonly administered medicines in order to act promptly in cases where side effects and adverse reactions occur.

Pharmacology

What medicines are

Medicines are made up of drugs, which are chemical compounds that are taken into the body to initiate a reaction in order to cause some sort of change to, or effect on, the body. The term 'medicines' and 'drugs' are often used interchangeably. However, it is important to note that a medicine may contain more than one drug or chemical compound, so a medicine can contain two or more drugs. These chemical compounds are made up of both natural and synthetic substances. Natural substances can come from a variety of sources, such as plants. Digoxin, a medicine used to treat **atrial fibrillation**, is extracted from the leaves of the digitalis plant. There is a whole host of herbal medicines available that are sourced from plants. Animal products are also used in medicines. Insulin obtained from the pancreas of pigs and cows is an example that, until fairly recently, was used in the treatment of **diabetes**. Now insulin is manufactured synthetically. Other natural sources used in medicines are derived from minerals and salts. Chloride and potassium are examples of such medicines. Synthetic medicines are those that are manufactured from man-made materials, mostly petrochemicals.

Typically, at least three names are applied to the same medicine. This is because medicines can be referred to by either their **chemical**, **generic** or **trade** (also referred to as **brand** or **proprietary**) **name**. The chemical name describes the molecular structure of the medicine. It is often only used during the developmental stages of the medicine. The generic name is a shorter version of the chemical name and the trade name refers to the title that the pharmaceutical company, who manufactured the medicine, gives it. The generic name is often the preferred method for prescribing medicines. This is because it more clearly indicates the class of the medicine and generic names are generally recognised internationally. The generic name tends to be more readily recognised by practitioners. For example, ibuprofen is a generic name for a **non-steroidal anti-inflammatory medicine (NSAID)** to treat pain associated with inflammation. Nurofen is an example of a popular NSAID. Nurofen is a brand name, but if you look at the ingredients that make up this medicine you will notice that ibuprofen is the main drug.

Medicines are also grouped into **classes** according to either their use or if they share similar characteristics. So, for example, paroxetine is the generic name given to a class of medicine that is termed a selective serotonin uptake inhibitor. Its chemical name is (3S, 4R)-3-(1, 3-benzodioxol-5-yloxymethyl)-4-(fluorophenyl) piperidine and its chemical structure is: $C_{19}H_{20}FNO_3$. Clearly, trying to recall the chemical compounds that make up this medicine would be very difficult. Imagine if you had to do this for all medicines! One of the main reasons why patients are prescribed this medicine is to treat the symptoms of depression. Seroxat is an example of one of the trade names of this medicine.

The use of medicines

Medicines are used to either treat or prevent a disease. When they are used for **therapeutic** (treatment) reasons, their purpose is to cure a disease, to reduce or improve the unpleasant symptoms a patient may be experiencing as a result of their disease, or to control the progression of a disease. For example, **antibiotics** may be administered to a patient who has a wound infection. The antibiotics will destroy or deactivate the bacteria present in the wound, thereby curing the wound infection. NSAIDs may be administered to a patient with **osteoarthritis** and will help to reduce inflammation and pain associated with this disease, thereby decreasing the amount of pain a patient will experience. Cytotoxic medicines may be administered to a patient with cancer to slow down the progression of the disease. They work by interfering with how cells are replicated, thus reducing the number of cancerous cells left in the body.

Medicines are also used for **prophylactic** reasons. When administered for this purpose the aim is to prevent a disease or a dangerous or unpleasant symptom of a disease from occurring. **Statins**, for example, are used to reduce **cholesterol** levels. High levels of cholesterol play a major role in the development of **heart disease** and **strokes**. It is thought that giving patients statins will reduce the development of such diseases. **Vaccines** are another example of medicines that are commonly given to prevent the development of diseases, such as mumps, measles or swine flu.

Medicines can also be used for diagnostic purposes. For example, **mydriatics** may be administered into the eye to facilitate the examination of the eye.

Activity 3.1   *Evidence-based practice and research*

Answer the following scenarios to test your understanding of medicines use. For each scenario decide what the medicine is used for, a reason why the patient may have been prescribed it and whether it has been prescribed for therapeutic or prophylactic reasons. You may wish to provide your answers in a table. You could use the following headings in your table: medicine, its use, why it is prescribed, prophylactic or therapeutic.

(a) Tia Hamilton is a nine-year-old girl who has recently emigrated from South Africa. She has been prescribed Bacillus Calmette-Guerin (BCG) vaccine.

(b) Rory Winters is a 45-year-old man. He has been prescribed paracetamol 1g as a once-only prescription.

(c) Jordan Black is a 28-year-old woman. She has been prescribed citalopram 20mg, to be administered once a day.

(d) Jacob Rogers is a 65-year-old man. He has been admitted to the ward for a left total knee replacement. He has been prescribed cefuroxime 1.5g IV for one dose and then 750mg for a further two doses only.

An outline answer is provided at the end of the chapter.

Pharmacokinetics

Pharmacokinetics is the study of what the body does to a medicine. It derives from the Greek words *pharmakon* (drug) and *kinetikos* (motion). It looks at how medicines are absorbed, distributed, metabolised and excreted from the body.

Absorption

The route of administration is the way the medicine enters your patient's body. The way that medicines are absorbed in the body initially depends on the route of administration. The most common route for administering medicines is by the oral route and most medicines that are taken orally are absorbed from the stomach, into the small intestine and then into the bloodstream. Due to the relatively fast emptying time of the stomach, many medicines will initially pass through the stomach before they are absorbed. It is in the small intestine that most absorption of oral medicines occurs.

Medicines can also be administered by the intravenous route (directly into a vein), intramuscularly (into a muscle), subcutaneously (under the skin), transdermally or topically (through the skin). With these routes the medicine enters the bloodstream directly from the site of administration.

Other routes include sublingual (under the tongue), **buccal** (in the cheek) and **nasal** (via the nasal passages). With these routes the medicine is absorbed through the **oral mucosa** and **mucous membranes** that line the nasal passages.

Your patients may also take their medicines via inhalation (directly into the lungs), or the **aural** route (into the ears) and the **ocular** route (into the eyes). Medicines may also be given **rectally** (directly into the rectum), **vaginally** (into the vagina), **intrathecally** (directly into the central nervous system) and **intravesically** (directly into the bladder).

Activity 3.2   *Evidence-based practice and research*

Consider the patients you will be predominantly caring for during your nursing pro-gramme. Identify the advantages and disadvantages to your patients of receiving their medicines by the various routes available. You could do this in the form of a table.

An outline answer is provided at the end of the chapter.

The absorption process begins when the medicine is introduced into the body. It ends when the medicine reaches the circulatory system. In order to reach the circulatory system the medicine first needs to dissolve to enable it to cross a **cell membrane**. How a medicine dissolves once it enters the body depends on its route of administration and also the chemical compounds that make up that particular medicine. Cell membranes are able to absorb medicines by various processes:

- **passive diffusion**;
- **facilitated diffusion** (also known as **facilitated transport**);
- **active transport**.

Before you continue reading this chapter, you may find it useful to refresh your understanding of **cell physiology**, to which the processes involved in absorption relate. Medicines that can **ionise** in solution will be unable easily to cross the cell membrane. Un-ionised medicines will find it far easier to cross the cell membrane. The process of ionisation will be explained in more detail later in the chapter.

Passive diffusion

Passive diffusion occurs when the concentration of the medicine on one side of the cell mem-brane is greater than that on the other side of the cell membrane. The medicine will move along a **concentration gradient** through the cell membrane to the area where there is less concentration of the medicine. This process does not require any energy; it is purely driven by the concentration gradient. (Imagine you parked your car on the top of a steep slope and took the handbrake off. The car would roll down the slope, even with the engine switched off.) This process will occur more quickly if the medicine molecules are small, soluble in water and are **lipids**.

Facilitated diffusion

Facilitated diffusion requires **carrier proteins** to move a medicine molecule across a cell membrane. The process still involves a medicine moving along a concentration gradient, to enable a higher concentration of the medicine to cross the cell membrane to the lower concentration. The carrier protein **binds** with the medicine molecule to move it across the cell membrane. (Imagine you needed to get the car back up the hill. The car would need to be filled with petrol in order for you to be able to turn on the ignition and drive it back up.)

Active transport

Active transport requires energy to move a medicine molecule across a cell membrane. With this process medicine molecules are pumped across the cell membrane, against a concentration gradient. The energy required is in the form of **adenosine triphosphate (ATP)**. This form of absorption will occur in cases where medicine molecules are too large to cross the cell membrane or they are moving against a concentration gradient. (Imagine you had to push the car back up the steep hill. You would need a lot of energy in the form of physical strength to enable you to do this.)

Ionisation of medicines

As already discussed, some medicine molecules require a form of energy in order to cross a cell membrane and enter the cell. We have discussed the forms of energy required for facilitated diffusion (carrier proteins) and active transport (such as ATP to pump the medicine molecules into the cell). The environment inside a cell is more acidic than outside, with the exception of cells lining the stomach. Referring to basic cell physiology, we know that molecules comprise two or more **atoms**. Atoms are electrically neutral, whereby they comprise negatively charged **electrons** and positively charged **protons**. When atoms lose or gain an electrical charge they become **ions**. Ions carry an electrical charge that enables them to move across cell membranes. There are factors that affect this process. For example, a very acidic environment such as the stomach (where medicines are absorbed when given via the oral route) will suppress the electrical charge of a medicine with a weak acid base such as aspirin (acetic acid). In this case the atoms that make up the medicine molecule will cross the cell membrane and enter the cell. Therefore a medicine with similar properties to aspirin will be absorbed mainly in the stomach. Many medicines have weak acid bases and thus, if administered via the oral route, will be absorbed largely in the stomach and small intestine.

Activity 3.3   *Evidence-based practice and research*

For each route of administration, list one commonly used medicine.

An outline answer is provided at the end of the chapter.

Distribution

Once a medicine has crossed the cell membrane and entered the circulatory system, it is distributed to the body tissues. Ideally, we would only want the medicine to target a specific tissue. For example, if a patient was administered gliclazide, to regulate their blood glucose levels, we would want it to selectively target the pancreas, which is the organ responsible for insulin production, which assists in regulating blood glucose levels. However, once a medicine enters the circulatory system it will travel to all parts of the body. Where it travels is dependent on whether it is a water-soluble or fat-soluble medicine. Medicines that are water soluble will stay in the circulating blood and also in the fluid surrounding the cells (**interstitial space**). Medicines that are fat soluble will target fatty tissues. This may offer an explanation as to why side effects are common with many medicines. Body tissues that are highly vascularised will receive the medicine before less well-vascularised areas. Like absorption, there are several factors that affect how a medicine is distributed.

Blood–brain barrier

Many medicines are unable to enter the brain due to a barrier between the brain and the circulatory system. This is commonly known as the blood–brain barrier. The barrier is comprised of a membrane that separates the circulating blood and **cerebrospinal fluid (CSF)**. It was discovered about a hundred years ago during an experiment where staining was carried out. Dye was injected into animals and was taken up in all body tissues except the brain. A further study a few years later, where dye was injected into the cerebrospinal fluids of animals, showed the uptake of dye in the cerebrospinal fluid only. The blood–brain barrier was later confirmed in the 1960s with the introduction of the scanning electron microscope. Its mechanism is primarily to protect the brain from harmful substances such as bacteria and from hormones and neuro-transmitters that are found elsewhere in the body. Only some medicines, made up of very small molecules, are able to cross this barrier. Consequently, this could prove problematic when trying to administer medicines that need to be delivered to the brain.

Metabolism

Metabolism is a process whereby the medicine is converted from one chemical compound into another. This is enabled by enzymatic activity. The processes involved will convert the medicine into a water-soluble form to make it easier to be excreted from the body. The main organ in the body where metabolism takes place is the liver. Metabolism has an effect on the **bioavailability** of a medicine. Bioavailability refers to the amount of the medicine that is left unchanged that is able to reach the circulatory system. It is important to know this, since medicine dosages will be prescribed according to the bioavailability of the medicine. The amount of medicine left unchanged can be influenced by a process called the **first pass effect** or first pass metabolism.

First pass effect

The first pass effect, also known as first pass metabolism, begins during the absorption process of a medicine, but it also influences the distribution of the medicine. All medicines that are absorbed from the gastrointestinal tract pass into the **portal blood system**. This part of the circulatory system transports the absorbed molecules of the medicine via the portal vein to the liver before the medicine is distributed to various parts of the body. The liver metabolises a large proportion of the medicine into **metabolites**. With some medicines so many metabolites are lost or **deactivated** during this process that only a small amount of the active medicine remains, which can then pass into the blood circulation and on to the rest of the body. This is known as the first pass effect. This explains why many medicines that are absorbed via the gastrointestinal system are administered to patients in higher doses than those given via alternative routes.

Activity 3.4   *Evidence-based practice and research*

Medicines administered by the intravenous route have 100 per cent bioavailability.

(a) What does this mean?
(b) Why does this happen?

An outline answer is provided at the end of the chapter.

Plasma protein binding

Most medicines bind to proteins as they flow through the body. The binding (or the bound medicine) does not produce any physiological effect. Only the unbound or free medicine is available to the tissues to exert a therapeutic effect. Certain medicines are more highly bound to proteins than others. These medicines need to be administered in higher doses to bring about a therapeutic effect. This is because there is less of the free medicine available in the circulatory system to reach the tissues, and also highly bound medicines are released more slowly into the circulatory system. Aspirin is an example of a medicine highly bound to the protein albumin. Several factors impact on the binding process. Aspirin and warfarin bind to the same protein, since both medicines have **anticoagulant** properties; it is often the case that the same or similar classes of medicines will compete for the same protein. If both medicines are administered at the same time, warfarin will be displaced. There will be higher levels of warfarin in the circulatory system. A reduction in plasma protein levels seen in malnourished patients and older adults will also have an effect on the action of a highly bound medicine.

Excretion

Excretion is the final process involved in pharmacokinetics and is the process involved in removing the medicine or its residue from the body. Medicines are excreted via several routes, the most common being via the kidneys (excreted in urine). Other routes of excretion include the gastrointestinal tract (excreted in faeces), the skin (excreted in sweat) and the lungs (excreted during exhalation of breath).

The rate of excretion is important as it determines the duration of action of the medication. Medicines that have been made water soluble by metabolism in the liver are easily excreted via the kidneys by a process known as **glomerular filtration**. Some medicines are reabsorbed through the **renal tubules** of the kidney by active transport (see the section on absorption on pp71–2).

Half-life (*t* 1/2)

The half-life of a medicine refers to the length of time it takes for the medicine to leave the body and leave one half of it remaining in the circulatory system. The half-life of a medicine is measured by the amount of medicine remaining in plasma. It is based on the plasma levels of a healthy individual. How quickly a medicine is eliminated from the body depends on several factors. For example, it can be excreted from the body, or moved to another body compartment such as intracellular fluid. The medicine can also be destroyed in the blood. Plasma protein binding, as discussed earlier, also has an effect on the half-life of a medicine. For example, highly bound medicines have a longer half-life than unbound medicines. This is because they remain in the body longer and release their active ingredient more slowly. The symbol *t* 1/2 is used to refer to the plasma half-life of a medicine.

To measure the half-life of a medicine, a dose is given to a patient (usually in a clinical trial). Blood samples are then taken at intervals and the results of the samples are plotted on a graph. Initially, the concentration levels of the medicine in the blood will be high and will gradually decline as the medicine is absorbed from its site of entry, distributed to its site of action, metabolised in the liver and finally excreted from the body. Figure 3.1 shows how the plasma levels of a medicine administered by the intravenous route (where rapid absorption into the circulatory system occurs) may look if the blood levels were plotted on a graph.

It is important to know the half-life since this will determine how much of a medicine should be given and also how frequently it should be administered. It is important to remember that various factors will affect the half-life of a medicine. For example, poor renal function in an older adult may result in the medicine taking longer to be excreted from the body. The half-life of a medicine is usually calculated during the trial or testing stages of a new medicine. This will be done before the medicine is made available for use on patients.

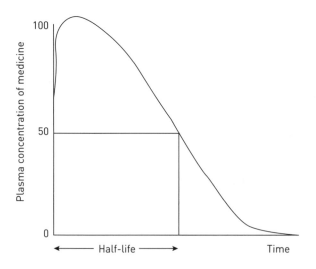

Figure 3.1: Plasma concentration levels and half-life of a medicine after a single dose administered via intravenous injection

Activity 3.5   *Evidence-based practice and research*

Tom Reynolds is a 46-year-old man. He has recently been diagnosed with schizophrenia. He has commenced treatment for his condition and has been prescribed flupentixol 12mg daily, which is an antipsychotic medicine. It has a half-life of approximately 20 hours.

Approximately how much of the medicine would remain in Tom's circulatory system after 20 hours?

Answers are provided at the end of the chapter.

Therapeutic range

In order to ensure a medicine is present in a sufficient concentration to have a desirable effect, without side effects, ideally the medicine should be present at a therapeutic level. Too much of a medicine will produce undesirable effects and too little will produce little therapeutic effect. Sometimes it is necessary to administer a **loading dose** of the medicine in order for it to be effective and to quickly bring the medicine into the therapeutic range. Smaller, regular maintenance doses are then administered to ensure the medicine stays within the therapeutic range in the blood.

Figure 3.2 demonstrates the concept of a therapeutic range. In this diagram you can see that a loading dose of a medicine has been administered. It quickly reaches and surpasses the ideal range for the medicine to be at its most effective. At this stage the patient may experience some unpleasant or even toxic effects of the medicine. The plasma concentration of the medicine then falls and it is at this stage that the medicine is unlikely to be effective. Subsequent doses of the medicine are given (we can see this from the peaks in the lines). These doses are called maintenance doses and are usually smaller than the initial loading dose. Once again we can see the peaks and troughs in the plasma concentration levels of the medicine. Ideally, we would want a medicine to stay in the therapeutic range for as long as possible as here it will give the patient the

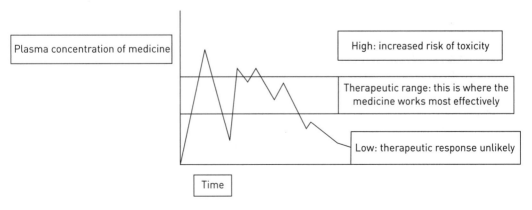

Figure 3.2: The therapeutic range of a medicine

most benefit and least side or toxic effects. This will be dependent on factors such as the strength of the dose given, the route of administration and the timing of the doses. Some medicines have very narrow therapeutic ranges and hence the patient needs close and regular monitoring of their plasma levels. Warfarin is one such example. Patients who are prescribed this medicine initially have their plasma concentration levels checked on a daily or alternate-day basis to determine the dose of warfarin they should be administered.

Factors affecting the pharmacokinetics of medicines

Routes of administration

As discussed earlier, there are several routes in which a medicine can be administered. The method by which a medicine enters the body plays a major role in the absorption process. For example, when taken via the oral route medicines are subjected to an acidic environment in the stomach that breaks down the chemical compound of the medicine. With many medicines taken via this route, much of the active ingredient is deactivated by this acidity and subsequently lost to the circulatory system. If food is present, stomach acidity is higher and it takes longer for the stomach to empty. Consequently, any medicines ingested will be subjected to a higher acidic environment for longer. This can be further exacerbated by the presence of certain foods in the stomach that can increase stomach acidity. Examples include protein products and alcohol. Some medicines will also affect the rate at which the stomach empties. For example, metoclopramide, a medicine commonly used to treat nausea and vomiting, increases the rate at which the stomach empties. This in turn will increase the rate of absorption. If several medicines are taken at the same time, some may be absorbed more quickly or more slowly than intended. Other routes that also result in a medicine entering the stomach include **enteral** routes such as via **nasogastric** or **gastrostomy** tubes.

The intravenous route for administration results in all of the medicine reaching the circulatory system. This is because medicines administered via this route are not absorbed in the stomach and are not subjected to the stage of first pass effect (see pp74–5), where much of a medicine is deactivated in the liver. This is why intravenous doses of a medicine are usually lower than when given via the oral route.

The rate of absorption of a medicine given via the intramuscular route is dependent on which muscle the medicine is injected into. Blood flow to the muscle will also be a factor in how much of the medicine is absorbed into the muscle. If the muscle is cold, the blood vessels will **vasoconstrict**, thus decreasing absorption. If the muscle is warm (for example, through exercise), then blood vessels will **vasodilate** and the absorption rate will be increased. Similar to the intravenous route, medicines administered in this way will bypass the stomach and the first pass effect in the liver.

The subcutaneous route for injecting medicines is another common route to use. The medicine is injected under the top two layers of skin. The absorption rate is considerably slower when compared to the intravenous or intramuscular route because the medicine has to pass through the fatty layers under the skin and then be absorbed into the circulatory system. Once again, the stomach and first pass effect are bypassed. Like muscle, the skin is affected by heat and cold, which in turn will affect the absorption rate of the medicine.

Medicines administered rectally or vaginally are usually in the form of **suppositories**, **pessaries**, liquids or creams. They are absorbed into the lining of the rectum or vagina and are then absorbed into the bloodstream. This method also bypasses the stomach and liver.

Sublingual or buccal administration results in the medicine being absorbed through the mucous membranes under the tongue or in the cheek. Similarly, if the nasal route is used, the medicine can be absorbed directly through the mucous membranes that line the nose. Some medicines will also be absorbed from the nasal mucosa and into the CSF (see the section on the blood–brain barrier on p74), thus exerting an effect on the brain. Absorption is often quicker than with the oral route since the medicine is able to directly enter the circulatory system. Only the **enzymes** present in saliva may deactivate some of the medicine, but these effects are much less when compared to those of the first pass effect.

The transdermal or topical route enables a medicine to be absorbed into the skin. As with the subcutaneous injection, this method is slow and the absorption rate is affected by heat or cold, due to the effects of vasoconstriction or vasodilation of the capillaries.

The ocular route enables a medicine to be absorbed through the cornea and conjunctiva of the eye to produce a local effect, while the aural route is used where a local effect of the medicine is required in the ear. Ointments, for example, would be administered directly into the ear.

Inhalation routes are used when a medicine needs to go directly into the lungs or other parts of the respiratory system. Smaller molecules of a medicine will be able to diffuse into the lungs and into the **alveoli**. Larger molecules of medicine may only be absorbed and diffused into the **bronchioles**.

Using the intravesical route enables a medicine to be administered directly into the bladder. Absorption of the medicine will have a local effect, that is, directly at the intended site. Superficial bladder tumours are commonly treated via intravesical medicines. There is a risk, however, that some of the medicine will be absorbed into the circulatory system and subsequently may have a systemic effect.

The intrathecal route enables a medicine to be administered directly into the intrathecal space surrounding the spinal cord. The medicine is injected into CSF to enable it to work on the central nervous system (CNS). This route will bypass the blood–brain barrier.

Age

Children's bodies are fundamentally different from those of adults, so there will be several differences to how their bodies deal with medicines. For example, children have less fat and muscle mass, so medicines delivered by the topical or subcutaneous route may have faster absorption rates. In the early stages of life the liver is less effective at metabolising medicines. The kidneys are also less able to excrete medicines in the first six weeks or so of life. The ageing process itself does not have an effect on the absorption of medicines. However, older adults may have underlying health conditions that impact on absorption rates. For example, if they have a gastrointestinal disease this may affect how the medicine is absorbed in the stomach. Older adults may also be taking several medicines at a time, some of which may interfere with the absorption of other medicines. Older adults have less **albumin** (a protein) in their blood. Therefore, less of the medicine undergoes protein binding and so more of the medicine is in the circulating blood and tissues. As a higher concentration of the medicine is present, this will produce an increased pharmacological effect. Enzymatic activity in the liver lessens with advancing age and this can lead to medicines not being metabolised, which again will cause increased levels of the medicine in the body. These increased levels could be dangerous to the patient. Medicines may also accumulate in the body due to a decrease in renal function, where medicines are not able to be fully excreted in the urine.

Size and body weight

Patients who are heavier may need larger doses of a medicine to bring about the desired effect. This is because they have more body tissue to absorb the medicine. Depending on the route of administration, this will also impact on the absorption of the medicine. For example, a medicine administered via the subcutaneous route will be absorbed much more slowly in a patient with excess adipose fat.

Gender

Physical differences between men and women will also affect absorption of medicines. For example, women have more fat cells than men and for medicines that deposit in fat the absorption rate will be slower.

Ethnicity/genetics

It is also known that genetic factors play a role in how a medicine works. For example, Herceptin, a medicine used in the treatment of breast cancer, is only effective for patients who have a particular **receptor** called human epidermal growth factor receptor 2 (HER2) in their genetic make-up. Some ethnicities are found to have higher rates of enzymatic activity in the liver than others and are therefore able to metabolise medicines more quickly. Those who have faster rates are known as fast **acetylators** and those with slower rates are called slow acetylators.

Nutritional status

Malnutrition (which includes anorexia and obesity) can affect how a medicine is absorbed. Anorexic patients have less body mass, which leads to less fat and muscle and fewer proteins. Medicine molecules need to bind with proteins to assist in the delivery of the medicine to its site of action. Obese patients have larger fat deposits and this may affect how some medicines are absorbed.

Medical conditions

There are numerous medical conditions that will impact on the absorption rate of medicines. These conditions are largely focused on the gastrointestinal system. For example, if a patient has diarrhoea, the absorption process will be speeded up as bowel motility is increased. Similarly, if a patient has undergone a bowel resection, part of the bowel used for absorption is no longer there. This may result in some or even all of the medicine not being absorbed.

Medicine product

Some medicines are designed to be absorbed more slowly than others. To stop them from being absorbed too quickly, they will be manufactured with an **enteric coated shell**, which is a protective cover that is able to resist breakdown by the stomach enzymes. The cover is designed to start disintegrating once the medicine enters the small intestine, which is less acidic than the stomach.

Psychological factors

How a patient feels about their medicine may also impact on how it actually works. If a patient believes that their medicine is beneficial to them, it is more likely to be effective. This is known as the **placebo** effect – *placebo* is Latin for 'I will please'. It is thought that physiological processes occur in the body that bring about a desired effect when the medicine is taken. For example, if morphine is given to a patient, the brain will release its own **endogenous** substances (natural pain killers) and the effect of the morphine in relieving the patient's pain may be greater than if the patient believed it would not help to reduce their pain. The use of placebos will be discussed in more detail in Chapter 4.

Pharmacodynamics

Pharmacodynamics is concerned with the effects a medicine has on the body. Ideally, we would want a medicine to act just enough to produce the desired effect. Unfortunately, side effects are often seen with many medicines. This is partly due to the chemical structure of the medicine and how the body is able to deal with it. The premise of pharmacodynamics is that a medicine is only able to work provided it stimulates a reaction with a living organism. The action of a particular medicine is dependent on proteins. These are present in the body in the form of receptors, enzymes and **ion channels**.

Receptors

It is thought that medicines may act at specific areas either on the cell membrane or within the cell. These specific areas are termed as receptors, which are proteins. These receptors react with certain chemicals in the body such as **hormones** and **neurotransmitters** to influence cell activity. Medicines that target receptors are called **agonists** or **antagonists**. Medicines bind with such receptors to either stimulate or prevent a response. Medicines that stimulate a response are termed as agonists and those that prevent a response are termed antagonists. Any chemical that binds to a protein receptor is termed a **ligand**. Receptors also have two properties – **specificity** and **affinity** (see below) – and medicines are designed to fit a receptor that can recognise it. Receptors are three-dimensional structures that will only allow a medicine that fits it exactly to attach (a bit like a key in a lock). The actions of a medicine are largely affected by how much of the medicine reaches a receptor and whether there is affinity (attraction) between the medicine and the receptor on the cell wall.

Agonists

Agonist medicines bind to receptors to bring about a physiological response. An example is insulin. If a patient is administered this medicine it will bind to specific insulin receptors to change the **permeability** of the cell membrane. This will enable glucose to move into the cell. Insulin is the hormone responsible for controlling the levels of glucose in the blood. As the dose of the agonist increases, the number of receptors activated also increases, thereby increasing the amount of insulin and the consequential effects on blood glucose levels. The amount of medicine administered will eventually reach a threshold where all the relevant receptors will be activated and there will be no more effect from the medicine. This is the reason why medicines are pre-scribed in a specific range of doses.

Antagonists

Antagonist medicines bind to receptors to prevent a physiological response. An example is diphenhydramine, which is an antihistamine used in the treatment of allergies. This medicine will bind to a histamine receptor to block the production of histamine. Therefore, physiological reactions associated with allergic reactions such as swelling or even anaphylaxis (see Chapter 5) will subside or be prevented from occurring. Like agonists, once a dose threshold has been reached there will be no more receptors to block. If increased doses of histamine are given, side effects will occur such as increased drowsiness.

Partial agonists

Partial agonists are medicines that are able to both stimulate and block a physiological response. How they work depends on the dosage of the medicine or the duration of its action. Its effects are less than those of agonists.

Affinity and specificity

Receptors are able to recognise specific chemical compounds present in the body, food and medicines. They will bind to these chemicals selectively. They also have the ability to bind tightly to certain chemicals they recognise. This means that the receptor has a high attraction or affinity to the chemical (in this case the medicine). The higher the affinity, the greater is the efficacy of the medicine and the lower the dose required to bring about a desired effect. Specificity means that some drugs can be designed specifically to bind with particular receptors.

Enzymes

Medicines can also exert their effect by disturbing the way in which enzymes act as catalysts for a variety of chemical reactions. Some medicines are termed **enzyme inhibitors** because they will bind to enzymes to decrease or stop the activity of a particular enzyme. For example, **ACE (angiotensin converting enzyme) inhibitors** such as enalapril, used to treat **hyper-tension**, work by inhibiting the conversion of angiotensin 1 to angiotensin 2. This prevents vasoconstriction of the blood vessels. It also inhibits the release of aldosterone, which subsequently causes less retention of sodium with a resultant fall in a patient's blood pressure. Other medicines work on enzymes to increase their activity. **Enzyme activators** are not as common as enzyme inhibitors.

Ion channels

Ions experience difficulty crossing cell membranes and entering cells. They therefore enter or leave cells via small pores created by ion channels. Ion channels can open or close in response to a stimulus, such as a medicine. Examples of medicines that will close an ion channel are **calcium channel blockers**, such as verapamil, which is used to slow down the heart rate.

Activity 3.6   *Evidence-based practice and research*

Refer back to the start of the chapter, where we met Mary Santini, the patient admitted to A & E after sustaining a fractured left neck of femur. Using the knowledge you have acquired, consider the pharmacodynamic and pharmacokinetic factors that may have contributed to Mary's death.

An outline answer is provided at the end of the chapter.

Chapter summary

This chapter has covered the basic principles of pharmacology. You should now understand how medicines affect the body (pharmacodynamics) and how medicines are absorbed, distributed, metabolised and excreted from the body (pharmacokinetics). Factors influencing these processes have also been discussed. Using this knowledge will enable you to have a better understanding of how the medicines you administer to your patients work. It should also help you to explain to your patients why they may experience some side effects with their medicines. Knowing your patients and understanding why medicines have to be taken as per instructed will ensure that side effects and adverse reactions are recognised, minimised and dealt with promptly. Completion of the activities will assist you in achieving the necessary proficiency for entry into your field of practice programme.

Activities: brief outline answers

Activity 3.1 Use of medicines (page 71)

Medicine	Its use	Why it is prescribed	Prophylactic or therapeutic?
BCG vaccine	Prevent development of tuberculosis (TB).	Mia has immigrated from a country where TB is prevalent.	Prophylactic
Paracetamol	Treatment of mild to moderate pain. Can also be used to reduce a high body temperature.	Rory may have a high temperature or he may have experienced pain.	Therapeutic
Citalopram	Treatment of depression or panic disorders.	The dose Jordan has been prescribed indicates that she is suffering from either depression or panic attacks.	Therapeutic
Cefuroxime	This is an antibiotic used in the treatment of, or to prevent, infection.	Jacob has been prescribed it to reduce the risk of him developing an infection post-operatively. If he was to develop an infection, this could impact on the viability of his artificial knee. The first dose is usually administered at the time of his anaesthetic, with the second dose administered 8 hours later and the third dose after 16 hours.	Prophylactic

Activity 3.2 Routes of administration (page 72)

Route	Advantages	Disadvantages
Intravenous	Quick administration; direct entry into circulation; rapid onset of action; no needles.	Requires peripheral cannula; risk of bloodstream infection.
Intramuscular	Quick administration; rapid onset of action.	Painful; needle phobias.
Subcutaneous	Quick administration.	Painful; needle phobias; slow onset of action.
Intrathecal	Quick administration; rapid onset of action; direct access to brain and nerves.	Painful; patient needs to keep very still during administration stage.
Intravesical	Local site of action; less likely to be unpleasant side effects associated with systemic action.	Urethral catheter required; invasive procedure; risk of urinary tract infections.
Transdermal/topical	Easy; self-application.	Messy; slow onset of action.

Rectal	Useful for those patients who are nil-by-mouth or suffering with nausea.	Slow onset of action; invasive procedure; may be uncomfortable.
Vagina	Local site of action; less likely to experience unpleasant side effects associated with systemic action.	Invasive procedure; may be uncomfortable; slow onset of action.
Oral	Easy; self-administration; medicine can be taken in a variety of different forms, e.g. tablets, liquids.	Tablets hard to swallow; unpleasant taste; difficulties with nausea and vomiting.
Sublingual/buccal	Easy; self-administration.	Unpleasant taste; patient needs education regarding not swallowing medicine.
Nasal	Easy; self-administration.	Irritant to nasal passages; unpleasant taste.
Inhalation	Easy; self-administration.	May leave unpleasant taste; good technique required.
Aural/ocular	Local site of action only.	Precision required for application of medicine.

Activity 3.3 Medicines for different routes (page 73)

There is a whole host of medicines that are administered by the various routes. The table below lists only a few. Please refer to a BNF for your particular patient group.

Route	Medicine
Intravenous	Benzylpenicillin
Intramuscular	Haloperidol
Subcutaneous	Heparin
Intrathecal	Bupivacaine
Intravesical	Doxorubicin
Transdermal/topical	Hydrocortisone
Rectal	Diclofenac
Vagina	Clotrimazole
Oral	Paracetamol
Sublingual/buccal	Glyceryl Trinitrate
Nasal	Ephedrine Hydrochloride
Inhalation	Salbutamol
Aural	Neomycin Sulphate
Ocular	Pilocarpine

Activity 3.4 Bioavailability (page 75)

(a) This means that all of a medicine that is given by the intravenous route remains active when it enters the circulatory system.
(b) This happens because the absorption process is bypassed as the medicine enters directly into the bloodstream and does not go through the process of first pass effect or metabolism.

Activity 3.5 Half-life of medicines (page 77)

6mg

Activity 3.6 Pharmacodynamic and pharmacokinetic factors (page 83)

Mary may have had impaired renal function, due to her age and dehydration. This would impact on the kidneys' ability to excrete both the diclofenac and the lithium effectively. Lithium has a relatively long half-life of about 22 hours. Lithium is mainly absorbed in the gastrointestinal tract and only very small amounts of lithium are metabolised. Therefore, most of it is freely circulating in the blood. This half-life would be extended if Mary had renal impairment. Most lithium is excreted via the kidneys. Non-steroidal anti inflammatory medicines such as diclofenac slow down the excretion of lithium. This causes an increase of lithium levels in the blood. Toxicity of lithium can lead to relatively mild symptoms such as diarrhoea and vomiting, and to life-threatening conditions such as renal failure, coma and even death.

Knowledge review

Now that you've worked through the chapter, how would you rate your knowledge of the following topics?

	Good	Adequate	Poor
1. Principles of pharmacokinetics. 2. Principles of pharmacodynamics. 3. Factors affecting pharmacokinetics. 4. Reducing adverse reactions.			

Where you're not confident in your knowledge of a topic, what will you do next?

Further reading

Clancy, J and McVicar, A (2009) *Physiology and Anatomy for Nurses and Healthcare Practitioners: A homeostatic approach*, 3rd edition. London: Hodder Arnold.

This is a useful accompaniment to pharmacology. Section 2 of this book provides a comprehensive overview of cell physiology and cell metabolism, both of which play vital roles in the pharmacology of medicines.

Greenstein, B and Gould, D (2004) *Trounce's Clinical Pharmacology for Nurses*, 17th edition. Oxford: Elsevier.

This is an easy-to-read book focusing on the principles of pharmacology. It also explores the use of medicines in relation to body systems and classes of medicines.

Karch, AM (2008) *Focus on Nursing Pharmacology*, 4th edition. Philadelphia, PA: Lippincott Williams and Wilkins.

This is a comprehensive textbook featuring an introduction to pharmacology. It also discusses medicines in relation to body systems.

Useful websites

www.bnf.org/bnf

This is home to the online *British National Formulary* where information on clinical conditions, medicines and their preparations can be reviewed. Please note, user registration is required, although this is free of charge.

www.bnfc.org/bnfc

This provides access to the online *British National Formulary for Children* where information on clinical conditions, medicines and their preparations can be reviewed. Please note, user registration is required, although this is free of charge.

www.merck.com/mmhe

This site gives access to The Merck Manuals online medical library. It provides a very useful and easy-to-navigate resource covering material on pharmacodynamics and pharmacokinetics in depth. No registration or subscription is required.

Chapter 4
Alternative approaches to medicines in nursing

NMC Standards for Pre-registration Nursing Education

This chapter will address the following competencies:

Domain 1: Professional values

2. All nurses must practise in a holistic, non-judgemental, caring and sensitive manner that avoids assumptions; supports social inclusion; recognises and respects individual choice; and acknowledges diversity. Where necessary, they must challenge inequality, discrimination and exclusion from access to care.

4. All nurses must work in partnership with service users, carers, families, groups, communities and organisations. They must manage risk, and promote health and wellbeing while aiming to empower choices that promote self-care and safety.

6. All nurses must understand the roles and responsibilities of other health and social care professionals, and seek to work with them collaboratively for the benefit of all who need care.

Domain 2: Communication and interpersonal skills

2. All nurses must use a range of communication skills and technologies to support person-centred care and enhance quality and safety. They must ensure people receive all the information they need in a language and manner that allows them to make informed choices and share decision making. They must recognise when language interpretation or other communication support is needed and know how to obtain it.

Domain 3: Nursing practice and decision-making

4. All nurses must ascertain and respond to the physical, social and psychological needs of people, groups and communities. They must then plan, deliver and evaluate safe, competent, person-centred care in partnership with them, paying special attention to changing health needs during different life stages, including progressive illness and death, loss and bereavement.

6. All nurses must practise safely by being aware of the correct use, limitations and hazards of common interventions, including nursing activities, treatments, and the use of medical devices and equipment. Nurses must be able to evaluate their use, report any concerns promptly through appropriate channels and modify care where necessary to maintain safety. They must contribute to the collection of local and national data and formulation of policy on risks, hazards and adverse outcomes.

continued overleaf . . .

continued . . .

8. All nurses must provide educational support, facilitation skills and therapeutic nursing interventions to optimise health and wellbeing. They must promote self-care and management whenever possible, helping people to make choices about their healthcare needs, involving families and carers where appropriate, to maximise their ability to care for themselves.

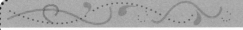

NMC Essential Skills Clusters

This chapter will address the following ESCs:

Cluster: Organisational aspects of care

9. People can trust the newly registered graduate nurse to treat them as partners and work with them to make a holistic and systematic assessment of their needs; to develop a personalised plan that is based on mutual understanding and respect for their individual situation, promoting health and well-being, minimising risk of harm and promoting their safety at all times.

10. People can trust the newly registered graduate nurse to deliver nursing interventions and evaluate their effectiveness against the agreed assessment and care plan.

20. People can trust the newly registered graduate nurse to select and manage medical devices safely.

By the first progression point:

1. Safely uses and disposes of medical devices under supervision and in keeping with local and national policy and understands reporting mechanisms relating to adverse incidents.

Cluster: Medicines management

34. People can trust the newly registered graduate nurse to work within legal and ethical frameworks that underpin safe and effective medicines management.

By the second progression point:

1. Demonstrates understanding of legal and ethical frameworks relating to safe administration of medicines in practice.

35. People can trust the newly registered graduate nurse to work as part of a team to offer holistic care and a range of treatment options of which medicines may form a part.

By the second progression point:

1. Demonstrates awareness of a range of commonly recognised approaches to managing symptoms, for example relaxation, distraction and lifestyle advice.
2. Discusses referral options.

continued overleaf . . .

continued . . .

40. People can trust the newly registered graduate nurse to work in partnership with people receiving medical treatments and their carers.

By the second progression point:

1. Under supervision involves people and carers in administration and self-administration of medicines.

Chapter aims

By the end of this chapter, you should be able to:

- identify the different types of alternative and complementary medicine;
- explain how psychological, cultural and religious factors influence patient choice in medicines management;
- gain an understanding of the health and safety aspects associated with the use of alternative and complementary therapies;
- discuss the implications associated with the use of medicines versus complementary and alternative medicines (CAMs);
- understand the application of non-pharmacological methods to treat pain.

Introduction

Case study

Ann, who was 30 years old and expecting her baby very soon, was informed that her baby was in the **breech** *position and that she would need to return to hospital in two weeks' time for a scan and* **external cephalic version**. *If this was unsuccessful a* **Caesarean section** *would be carried out. Ann desperately wanted to give birth naturally. She asked the midwife if there were any complementary and alternative therapies that she could use to improve the possibility of a natural birth. The midwife was dismissive of CAMs and informed Ann that such therapies would not help turn the baby and that Ann should expect to have a Caesarean section if the external cephalic version was unsuccessful in two weeks' time. Despite the midwife's assurance that CAMs do not work, Ann reviewed online literature and found that there were a number of things that she could try. She decided to try visualising the baby turning, tilting her pelvis, acupuncture and massage. At the scan two weeks later it was found that Ann's baby had turned into the vertex position. Ann was able to give birth naturally.*

This case study has shown that there is much we still do not understand about the workings of CAMs, and that practitioners and science need to keep an open mind about any benefits and pitfalls that they may have. We will return to this case study when we discuss nurses' roles and responsibilities in the administration of CAMs.

Da wearo he untrum on feferadle

Old English was by no means deficient in medical terms. The translation of the above quotation means 'then he became ill with a fever-disease'. Fumigation, which meant to burn incense, was known as a remedy for fever. This has since been refuted.

There were some treatments prescribed in the Old English medical treatises which sometimes, at least, failed to hinder recovery and sometimes even gave relief. The old folk remedy of using stinging nettles to treat the pain and swelling of rheumatic joints was probably based on the idea of treating like with like. Honey has a long history of over 4,000 years as a natural remedy in the field of wound care to **debride** and encourage new cell growth in healing wounds. There was an old method of using 'egg white and oxygen' in wounds. This went out of fashion some 20 years ago. In recent years honey and oxygen have enjoyed a revival, with considerable amounts of research being performed and adding to an existing body of evidence.

There has been a significant increase by both the general public and health professionals in the use of CAMs over the last two decades (Cramer et al., 2010). A CAM can be defined as *any health improving technique outside the mainstream of conventional medicine* (Ernst et al., 1995, p506). According to the World Health Organization (WHO, cited in Edirne et al., 2010), more than three-quarters of the world's population rely upon CAMs for healthcare. Healthcare professionals have a responsibility to review safe and reliable evidence that can be used to enable patients to make informed choices about their care. The health professional needs to be aware of contraindications between CAMs and traditional Western medicine. Concerns about the lack of evidence-based research underlying CAMs may have prevented healthcare professionals from advising patients on their safe use, but nurses are seen as reliable sources of information and they need to be able to educate patients on the potential benefits and side effects of various complementary and alternative treatments.

This chapter will discuss the different types of alternative and complementary medicines, including the health and safety aspects associated with the use of these therapies, highlight the arguments associated with the use of Western medicine versus CAMs, explain how psychological, cultural and religious factors influence patient choice, and discuss the application of non-pharmacological methods to treat pain.

Complementary and alternative medicines

Before we discuss the different types of alternative and complementary medicine we need to define CAMs, and review the relevant history.

What are complementary and alternative medicines?

Complementary and alternative medicines (CAMs) is a title used to refer to a diverse group of health-related therapies and disciplines that are not considered to be a part of mainstream medical care, and encompasses therapies with a historical or cultural, rather than a scientific, basis. The Cochrane Collaboration's definition of CAMs is:

> *a broad domain of healing resources that encompasses all health systems, modalities, and practices and their accompanying theories and beliefs other than those intrinsic to the politically dominant health systems of a particular society or culture in a given historical period.*

The philosophy of CAMs is fundamentally about **holism** and individualistic care. CAMs take into account the patient's psychosocial, physical and spiritual well-being. CAMs have a number of common characteristics, including a focus on individualised treatments, treating the whole person, promoting self-care and self-healing, and recognising the spiritual nature of each individual. Other terms sometimes used to describe CAMs include 'natural medicines', 'non-conventional medicines' and '**holistic** medicines'. However, CAM is currently the term used most often (House of Lords, 2000).

Activity 4.1   *Reflection*

List the complementary and alternative medicines that you are aware of.

As this activity is based on your own reflection, there is no outline answer at the end of the chapter.

You could have listed any of the hundreds of therapies currently practised in the UK. The House of Lords (2000) classified acupuncture, chiropractic, herbal medicine, homeopathy and osteopathy as alternative medicines and the Alexander technique, aromatherapy, Bach flower remedies, bodywork therapies (i.e. massage), reflexology, counselling, stress therapy, hypnotherapy and meditation as complementary therapies.

History of CAMs

CAMs are extremely diverse in their foundations and methodologies. Practices appear to incorporate or base themselves on folk knowledge, spiritual beliefs, traditional medicine or newly conceived approaches to healing.

In ancient times the use of herbs and other plant extracts, hands-on healing and ritualistic approaches were accepted forms of remedy for many health problems. Many healers during this time were women. The rise of Christianity during the Middle Ages called into question the role of the lay healer with the belief that only God could heal.

During the seventeenth century René Descartes, a French philosopher, suggested that ill health was the result of physical malfunction and introduced the scientific study of health and disease. The development of the biomedical approach in the West grew over the next two centuries as a result of this new-found scientific knowledge about the human body. Western medicine separates the body from the mind and developed as a discipline that seeks to understand and treat the body as a series of parts. It also seeks to identify symptoms and to prescribe the appropriate pharmacological substance or medical procedure in treatment. The introduction of the National Health Service (NHS) in the 1940s led to an increase in desirability of Western orthodox medicine. With the emergence of science-based medicine, based on clinical trials, the popularity of CAMs was reduced by the Western medical fraternity. Their main argument was that, because there had not been any clinical trials carried out on CAMs, it was impossible to prove the benefits these techniques offered to mankind.

An increasing number of people are becoming disenchanted with medical treatments that have been clinically tested, the results of which have appeared in medical journals. A rise in popularity of CAMs over the last few decades had been influenced by a rise in consumer knowledge and a lack of faith in the efficacy of some orthodox treatments.

To summarise, we have established that the term 'CAMs' covers a diverse group of health-related therapies. These therapies have been classified by the House of Lords into two broad categories. CAMs focus on individualisation, treating the whole person and promoting self-care, and these are underlying principles of nursing. CAMs have a long history but their benefits are being questioned by contemporary medicine.

CAMs versus Western medicine

The validity and efficacy of CAMs has been questioned by Western medical practitioners. The main arguments focus on the validity, efficacy of the CAMs, and the placebo effect. These arguments will be discussed below.

Activity 4.2   *Reflection*

Consider your own views of CAMs. Have you used any of them, and did they work?

As this activity is based on your own reflection, there is no outline answer at the end of the chapter.

In Activity 4.2 you may have listed a therapy that you have found beneficial. If this is the case, your opinion is not based on reading medical journals, but on first-hand experience. Remember that all your patients have such experiences, too.

Questioning the validity and efficacy of CAMs

The medical community has generally not accepted the claims made by complementary and alternative practitioners because an evidence-based assessment of the safety and **efficacy** of these practices was either not available or had not been performed until recently. Because CAMs tend to lack evidence, or may even have repeatedly failed in randomised controlled trials, they have been advocated as non-evidence-based medicines, or not medicines at all. Western medicine has likened CAMs to beliefs in the magic and superstition that medicine relied on before modern scientific advances. However, CAMs have characteristics commonly found in mainstream Western healthcare, such as a focus on good nutrition and preventive practices.

It is entirely possible that some of the remedies under the CAMs heading are ineffective or even dangerous, but that is not an appropriate reason to question the **validity** and efficacy of all complementary and alternative treatments entirely. To assert that all alternative remedies are ineffective because one such remedy was proven so is preposterous.

The idea that CAMs cannot be tested has begun to change. Researchers have started to conduct clinical trials on the testing of the more popular methods of treatment, such as acupuncture and holistic healing. If the safety and effectiveness of a CAM is ascertained it will become a mainstream medicine again and will no longer be 'alternative' or 'complementary' and may therefore become widely adopted by conventional practitioners.

The placebo effect in CAMs has often been used by Western medical practitioners to discredit the outcomes, but it is not just in CAMs that the placebo effect occurs. Drug trials using a sugar pill as a placebo to test the efficacy of new treatments yield placebo effects.

Placebo effects are non-specific effects on a treatment outcome, or effects that can happen in a clinical trial when a patient thinks they are receiving an intervention to test the efficacy of a particular treatment or therapy. The placebo effect accounts for about a third of the benefits of any treatment (Associated Press, 2009). This finding was supported during a trial of a new drug to relieve **lupus** symptoms, which found that 30 per cent of patients felt better when they received a placebo instead of the actual medication (Associated Press, 2009). Placebo effects in complementary medicine highlight the complexities involved in treating individuals, including the influence of 'human factors' and a 'therapeutic' setting on the care given.

The view of the medical community, however, seems to have had little impact on the growing popularity of CAMs among the general population. An increasing number of people in the UK have been turning to these treatments in addition to, or instead of, traditional Western medicines. Lorenc et al. (2009) estimate that 20–28 per cent of the UK population use CAMs. One argument for the acceptance of CAMs is the psychological impact they have on patients. Herbal treatments and acupuncture give people hope for the alleviation of their symptoms.

Cooperation between CAMs and Western medicine is known as **integrated medicine**. One example where Western medicine and CAMs were integrated is in the case of the television host Caron Keating. Caron was diagnosed with breast cancer and for seven years underwent both conventional and alternative treatments in the quest for a cure. Alternative treatments included acupuncture for pain management, reflexology, massage, and colonic irrigation. Unfortunately, despite her determination to beat breast cancer, Caron died.

It is important that you have an understanding of the arguments regarding the benefits and pitfalls of CAMs to enable you to review the literature with an open mind, and to ensure that you present an unbiased account when discussing the use of CAMs (in addition to, or instead of, traditional Western treatments) with your patients.

Overview of CAMs

It is valuable to have an understanding of the different CAMs, whether you are choosing for yourself or supporting a patient. A brief overview of various CAMs is given here, but you should have access to a source of good information on all therapies, examples of which are given at the end of the chapter.

Acupuncture

Acupuncture was first discovered around 4000BC, when it was noticed that non-fatal arrow wounds seemed to be linked to the disappearance of long-term health problems. There are two schools of thought about how acupuncture works. Some acupuncturists believe that health can only be balanced when the body is in **equilibrium**. If this balance is disturbed, this results in ill health. Other acupuncturists believe that acupuncture points correspond to nerve pathways, which, when activated by the insertion of a needle, release **endorphins** that in turn block impulses to the brain.

Acupuncture aims to restore a natural balance of health and involves the insertion of fine-gauged needles into the body over specific points to modify physiological function. It can be used in conjunction with electrical stimulation, heat or herbs. The WHO (cited in Edirne et al., 2010) suggests that acupuncture may be effective for patients with arthritis, back and muscle pain, sciatica, anxiety, depression, insomnia, asthma, bronchitis, common colds, tinnitus, headache, toothache, diarrhoea, constipation, menopausal symptoms, premenstrual syndrome, acute and chronic pain, chronic fatigue syndrome and addiction, including those who want to stop smoking.

Side effects of the therapy are rare, although there have been cases where a **pneumothorax** occurred when chest needles were inserted too deeply. Bleeding and infection can occur in the event of an improper insertion technique or poor decontamination procedures.

Alexander technique

The Alexander technique was first described in the late nineteenth century and focuses on changing the posture of the client in order to restore the natural curvature of the spine. Clients undertake a course consisting of approximately 20 30-minute sessions. The technique has been found to offer relief of backache, neck stiffness, asthma, peptic ulcers, hypertension, irritable bowel syndrome and repetitive strain injury.

Aromatherapy

Aromatherapy was first used in ancient Egypt in 3000BC and is the external use of essential oils that have been extracted from plant flowers, roots, seeds, berries or leaves, usually by distillation. The essential oils are applied directly on to the skin during massage, as a compress or via the lungs in vaporisers. Essential oils may have sedative, stimulatory, analgesic, antispasmodic or anti-bacterial effects.

Aromatherapy aims to enhance a feeling of 'wellbeing' and promotes emotional and physical good health. It has been documented that the use of the essential oil orange may provide relief of anxiety and the smell of peppermint may decrease post-operative nausea and vomiting. Aromatherapy may be used to treat anxiety, arthritis, asthma, colds, depression, digestive problems, hypertension, **insomnia**, migraines, muscular pain, nausea, premenstrual tension and stress.

Essential oils must be used cautiously during pregnancy or by people with epilepsy, high blood pressure or allergies. There is evidence that some vaporised oils can cause skin reactions, and some essential oils may cause **photosensitivity**.

Chiropractic

Spinal manipulation has existed since approximately 380BC. Chiropractors believe that, if the spine's mobility is compromised, a problem could arise elsewhere in the body. They therefore focus on the manipulation of the skeletal frame to correct the alignment of bones and joints to restore nerve function and alleviate pain in order to promote better physical body health. This technique has been successful in treating lower back pain, head, neck and upper body pain, rheumatism and migraines. Treatment is not advised if there is a history of inflammation, spinal tumours, circulatory problems or **aneurysms**.

Herbal medicine

There is evidence that herbal medicines have been in use since at least 1BC; however, archaeological findings have confirmed the use of herbal medicines many thousands of years earlier. Today, a large number of pharmaceutical preparations contain an active constituent extracted from plant sources; examples include digitalis (foxglove) and aspirin (willow and meadowsweet). Herbal medicine is especially effective in treating skin conditions, inflammation, migraines, and hormonal and gynaecological problems. Contraindications include ginseng, which should not be used by people with anxiety, tension or restlessness, and ginkgo, which, because of its anti-coagulation properties, should not be taken with aspirin, warfarin or heparin.

Activity 4.3   *Evidence-based practice and research*

Research information about the contraindications for St John's wort and liquorice.

An outline answer is provided at the end of the chapter.

As you learned from Activity 4.3, herbal medicines must be chosen carefully. In the next activity, you will find out about how herbal medicines can interact with prescription medicines.

Activity 4.4   *Evidence-based practice and research*

Interactions between herbal medicines and other prescribed medicines are possible. Document one example of where a drug interaction might occur.

An outline answer is provided at the end of the chapter.

As you learned from Activity 4.4, there are a number of possible interactions between herbal and prescribed medicines. Examples of these interactions are detailed in Table 4.1 (see page 106). It is important for nurses to be aware of these interactions to allow them to inform their patients in a bid to prevent these interactions occurring. In the next activity, you will find out about substances that patients need to be advised to avoid if they are undergoing homeopathic treatment.

Homeopathy

Homeopathy was first described in the eighteenth century and is based on the law of similars (let like be cured by like). Homeopathic medicines are produced from plants, metals, minerals, venoms, stings and bacteria. The original sources are diluted many times in a water and alcohol base. At each dilution the substance is shaken vigorously. Homeopaths believe that this process gives the final product its power to heal. Homeopathy can be used to assist with a large number of symptoms and conditions, including nausea, stress and wound healing. Contraindications include those found in patients who have diabetes and milk sensitivity. Although dismissed by many as 'unscientific', modern science is beginning to explain the principles behind homeopathy.

Activity 4.5   *Evidence-based practice and research*

What things are patients undertaking homeopathic treatment instructed to avoid?

An outline answer is provided at the end of the chapter.

As you learned from Activity 4.5, there are a few substances (e.g. coffee) that patients should be advised to avoid if they are undergoing homeopathic treatment, as these substances are thought to counteract the effect of the herbal medicine.

Humour/laughter therapy

The benefits of humour and laughter have long been recognised, but their therapeutic nature has only recently been identified. Humour and laughter have been shown to reduce anxiety, relieve pain and reduce muscle tension. Humour and laughter have also been shown to increase oxygen delivery to the tissues by increasing the rate and depth of breathing and the heart rate. When relaxation occurs, the patient often experiences a lowered heart rate and decreased blood pressure. Humour and laughter therapy can take many forms, including pictures and showing comedies.

Hypnosis

Hypnosis is an alternative state of consciousness where the patient's attention is focused away from reality. Therapists using this technique can help to bring about changes in the physical or emotional health of a patient, but only if that person is willing to be hypnotised. Hypnosis can be used for chronic, acute and procedural pain, asthma, childbirth, irritable bowel syndrome, smoking cessation and stress management. Hypnosis should not be used if an individual has severe depression, epilepsy or psychosis.

Massage

Massage has been performed since around 3000BC; however, during the Middle Ages religious dogma and superstition considered massage to be sinful because it was regarded as being physically and emotionally pleasurable. The rhythmic movement of massage has been found to be comforting and relaxing and has the following beneficial effects: reduced anxiety, relief of muscle tension, pain relief and improved local blood circulation. Massage is not recommended for patients with hypothermia, acute back pain, cardiovascular conditions, varicose veins, **lymphoma** and chronic fatigue syndrome.

Meditation

Meditation is used as a way of harnessing energy, power and control of the mind using only our own abilities to concentrate, focus and control our thoughts and emotions to calm and slow the body. Meditation is helpful for relaxation and in treating anxiety, insomnia, pain, phobias and post-traumatic stress disorder. There is a risk of orthostatic hypotension and patients should be advised to rise slowly from the sitting position.

Music therapy

Music therapy uses harmonic melody to diminish stress, pain and anxiety. There is evidence that shows that patients who are exposed to sedative music perioperatively have diminished analgesic medication requirements post-operatively.

Osteopathy

Osteopathy was founded in the late nineteenth century. Osteopaths believe that the musculoskeletal system is related to the autonomic nervous system, connecting the muscles, tendons and organs throughout the whole body. Osteopathy uses a 'hands-on' approach to ease pain, reduce swelling and improve mobility.

Prayer

Prayer is the common language of the faithful and is used to communicate with a higher power. Regular prayer can produce positive and reassuring effects within the individual, especially when he or she is faced with difficult or hopeless situations. Prayer may result in improved coping, increased relaxation and lowered blood pressure.

Reflexology

Reflexology has been used since approximately 2300BC. Reflexologists believe that reflexes exist in the feet and hands that correspond to the glands, organs and body parts. It is through these that vital energy flows. Therapists using reflexology apply pressure to specific pressure points on the soles of the feet to relax the patient and to enhance the function of various body organs. Reflexology has been shown to have psychological benefits, improve respiratory rates, decrease pain and anxiety, and reduce premenstrual tension. Reflexology should not be used on an inflamed foot or a foot that has an intravenous needle or cannula inserted.

Reiki

Reiki refers to a universal life energy that flows through all living things. It is a form of spiritual healing. Practitioners believe that, by moving energy through the body by the use of their hands, stress can be reduced and relaxation evoked. Reiki has been used in wound healing, pain management and stress reduction.

Therapeutic touch

The oldest written documentation of healing with touch is from 5,000 years ago. The aim of therapeutic touch is to rebalance the energy field of the patient to bring about relaxation and facilitate healing. Therapeutic touch has been shown to be effective for pain relief, anxiety, headaches, insomnia and hypertension.

Activity 4.6   *Communication*

You are working as a student nurse under the supervision of a practice nurse in a GP surgery and two patients ask your advice on the use of CAMs. Sheila, a mental health patient, suffers from insomnia and is thinking of using such a therapy.

• What information would you give Sheila?

James is a child with a learning disability. Each time he visits his GP he becomes extremely anxious. His mother asks you to explain what she could do to reduce his anxiety.

• What information would you give the mother?

Outline answers are provided at the end of the chapter.

As you learned from Activity 4.6, a nurse must give the person asking for advice non-biased information about CAMs to allow them to make an informed decision.

In summary, various CAMs have been introduced, the contraindications discussed and the potential benefits identified. It is important that nurses have a good understanding of these therapies so that they can provide evidence-based information for their patients from a non-biased viewpoint.

Factors affecting patient choice

There are a number of factors that may influence a person's choice to consult a CAM practitioner or to take part in such a therapy. The decision to use a CAM will be determined by social and psychological factors, in addition to considering the side effects of a particular CAM and the anticipated benefits of this medicine. Ethical, cultural, religious, and family and friend influences impacting on the use of CAMs will be considered.

Culture

Culturally, there appears to be a difference in the use of CAMs. Racial and ethnic differences in CAM use are generally attributed to cultural beliefs and practices. There is evidence that the use of CAMs is higher among women, non-Hispanic Whites, and those with poorer health status (Kronenberg et al., 2006). Factors such as education, income, access to resources and availability of healthcare play a prominent role in the use of CAMs. Studies based primarily on White populations indicate that CAM users tend to be well educated and more affluent. Yet studies in minority populations have found an inverse relationship between socioeconomic factors and use of some CAM modalities. Studies of Black Americans indicated that families in which the father had less than a high-school education were more likely to use home remedies than families in which the father had at least some college education. Similarly, herbal medicine among Mexican Americans has been associated with lower income and fewer years of education. However, Chao and Wade (2008) found that income was not associated with CAM use among Black or Chinese American women. This finding may have occurred because those people who are unable to afford US health insurance are probably unable to afford to pay for 'orthodox' medicine.

Locus of control

Locus of control refers to the extent to which individuals believe that they can control events that affect them (Lorenc et al., 2009).

Activity 4.7   *Reflection*

Do you believe that you control your own destiny or that your destiny is controlled by external forces (such as fate, a god or powerful others)? Consider how your views affect your use of healthcare, your choices and your view of outcomes. You could talk to relatives or friends with different points of view, and see how their mindsets affect their use of healthcare.

As this activity depends on your own views, there is no outline answer at the end of the chapter.

Individuals with a high internal locus of control believe that events result primarily from their own behaviour and actions. They have better control of their behaviour and are more likely to attempt to influence other people than those with a high external locus of control. Those with a high internal locus of control are also more likely to assume that their efforts will be successful. They are more active in seeking information and knowledge concerning their situation. Those with a low internal locus of control or a high external locus of control believe that powerful others, fate or chance primarily determine events.

In other words, people whose locus is internal believe that they control their lives. People whose locus is external believe that their environment, some higher power or other people control their decisions and their lives. Most people fall between these two extremes.

Religion/spirituality

Few topics generate more disagreement than the relationship between religion and health. Consensus seems to be that some patients draw on prayer and meditation to navigate and overcome the spiritual challenges that arise in their experiences of illness. It is believed that religion and spirituality help people to find meaning and value in their experience of illness. The decision to seek out CAM practitioners may be initiated by a sense of desperation, or by a pull towards an alternative ideology. Thus, CAMs that offer people a way to tap into spiritual energies have become very appealing.

Influence of family and friends

Case study

David has a history of back pain. He has tried using hot-water bottles to relieve the pain as well as painkillers. David does not like taking painkillers because of their potential side effects, and the hot-water bottles do not have a lasting effect. During conversations with friends and family, several CAMs have been recommended. David researches these recommendations online. He decides that osteopathy may help him. After five treatments David has found that his pain is controlled.

Friends and family may be involved in decisions regarding the use of CAMs. They may either help the patient move towards making a decision, or make the decision for the patient. Decisions about CAMs for children tend to be made by the parents of the child; in the main, the mother makes this decision (Lorenc et al., 2009). The Children Act 1989 (DH, 1997a) empowers the parent to take responsibility for making decisions about medical treatment on the child's behalf. However, it is possible for a child to consent at any age if they are assessed as having the necessary capacity to consent to medical examination and treatment. This is known as Gillick competence. By the age of 16 a child has the right to consent to medical examination and treatment by statute (Griffith and Tengnah, 2010).

In summary, some of the main influences surrounding the decision to use CAMs have been addressed. These influences come from many sources, including self, religion, and friends and family. Nurses need to be mindful of these influences and to respect decisions made by their patients.

Pain management

Pain management is a process of providing care that alleviates or reduces pain and this can sometimes be very challenging.

Gate control theory

The gate control theory was first proposed in 1965 by Melzack and Wall. According to the gate control theory of pain, our thoughts, beliefs and emotions affect how much pain we feel from a given physical sensation. The fundamental basis for this theory is the belief that psychological as well as physical factors guide the brain's interpretation of painful sensations and the subsequent response.

Melzack and Wall (1965) suggested that a 'gating system' existed in the central nervous system that opens and closes to let pain messages through to the brain or to block them. First, sensory messages travel from stimulated receptors (**thermoreceptors** and **nociceptors**) to the spinal cord via **afferent nerve** pathways. Sharp, pricking pain sensations are conducted by **myelinated** axons and aching, throbbing pain sensations are conducted by non-myelinated axons. The gating mechanism exists within the dorsal horn of the spinal cord. The pain impulses have to reach a certain threshold to force the gate to open. Pain receptors **synapse** with projection cells, which go up the spinothalamic tract to the thalamus, and to inhibitory **interneurons** within the dorsal horn. Once the sensory message reaches the brain, the information is processed in the context of the individual's current mood, state of attention and prior experience. The integration of all of this information influences the perception and experience of pain, and guides the individual's response. Descending fibres synapse in the dorsal horn and can modify the transmission of pain signals. Either the inhibitory interneurons will be activated and pain signals are blocked and lower amounts of pain are experienced, or the pain gates in the dorsal horn will be stimulated to open wider, the pain signal intensifies and pain will increase.

Factors associated with the experience of pain

There is evidence that psychological and social factors influence an individual's experience of pain.

Despite numerous research studies looking at gender differences in pain, the findings have been unequivocal. There is therefore no evidence to support a consistent pattern of pain appreciation in males and females. The literature addressing the influence of age on pain is also not straightforward. It has been suggested that ageing is associated with enhanced analgesia, indicating that older people require less analgesia to obtain effective relief. However, it has also been argued that older people under-report the amount of pain they experience. Culture appears to influence an individual's expression of pain. People from Latin origins tend to be more expressive about their pain compared to the White Anglo-British population (Thomas, 2007). Pain may be tolerated better by different ethnic groups. African Americans reported greater levels of pain than White Americans for certain conditions (Edwards et al., 2001).

Emotion can influence an individual's pain experience and there is an association between pain and anxiety. There is evidence that if the anxiety level is high this correlates to an increased perception of pain. Being in pain can lead to a low mood, depression and feelings of worthlessness (Eccleston et al., 2003). In addition, it has been found that people who are depressed experience more severe pain (Carr et al., 2005).

Pain is a personal experience and no one else can ever really know anyone else's experience of pain. Therefore, it has been accepted that the amount of suffering can only be assessed accurately by patients themselves. There is a large number of ways that pain can be assessed; these include visual analogue scales, numerical rating scales, simple descriptor scales and picture scales.

Use of analgesics in pain management

Pain can be treated with analgesics. Analgesics have been divided into two broad groups: anti-inflammatory and **opioids**.

Anti-inflammatory analgesics act on the peripheral site and include paracetamol and aspirin. Paracetamol can cause liver damage in an overdose, but is safe in normal dosage. Aspirin has many contraindications that relate primarily to its thrombotic regulation. Non-steroidal anti-inflammatory drugs (NSAIDs) are used to treat inflammation as well as pain, but are contra-indicated in patients with renal impairment and asthma. One example of a NSAID is ibuprofen. Ibuprofen is an over-the-counter drug and is known to have an anti-platelet effect.

Opioid analgesics include codeine, dihydrocodeine, dextropropoxyphene, morphine and dia-morphine. These drugs can cause nausea, vomiting and constipation. and may cause respiratory depression. Pethidine, fentanyl and alfentanil can be given as alternatives to morphine. Fentanyl appears to have the least number of side effects.

Alternative methods used to relieve pain

In addition, or as an alternative to the use of analgesia, CAMs may help to reduce or alleviate pain.

Distraction

Distraction therapy is a technique in which sensory stimuli are provided to patients in order to divert their attention from an unpleasant experience, such as pain. The use of nature scenes and sounds has been shown to be an effective tool for distraction.

Relaxation and visualisation

Relaxation aims to bring the mind to a state of balance and peace. The individual can either tense and relax successive groups of muscles or, in a quiet environment, repeat a word or phrase over and over again in order to disregard everyday thoughts and to promote a state of well-being. Relaxation appears to be an effective treatment because it reduces muscle tension and fear associated with the anticipation of pain. Visualisation is the use of mental imaging to alleviate and prevent disease. The individual is taught to focus on an appropriate image to induce a feeling of peace or happiness, or to promote beneficial changes in health or circumstance. Imagery using multiple senses can be useful in pain management.

Transcutaneous electrical nerve stimulation (TENS)

A TENS machine is a small battery-operated pack that generates impulses via electrodes. The electrodes produce continuous low-intensity electrical pulses to the skin. TENS stimulates the large myelinated fibres, which simultaneously closes the gate (situated in the dorsal horn of the spinal cord) on the smaller non-myelinated fibres, thus reducing pain. The frequency and duration of the pulses can be varied by the patient, who raises the strength of stimulation until a comfortable tingling is felt in the area supplied by the nerve that is being stimulated. TENS is a widely used non-invasive method of pain relief during the early labour of childbirth in the UK (Moore et al., 1997).

Activity 4.8   *Communication*

Reena has terminal cancer and is constantly feeling pain. She is thinking of using alternative therapies instead of Western medicine. What information would you give Reena?

An outline answer is provided at the end of the chapter.

Activity 4.8 reiterates the importance of giving non-biased information to your patients. It is important that you explain that CAMs can be used alongside conventional treatments for pain and discuss the possible contraindications of both CAMs and analgesia.

It is important for nurses to have an understanding of the theory of pain and to be aware of factors that affect pain. This understanding should help you to empathise with the patient's pain experience. Once you understand both conventional medicine and CAMs, you can provide patients with information to help them make informed choices about their pain control.

Over-the-counter medicines and home remedies

Home remedies and over-the-counter medicines are used by a large proportion of the UK population.

Over-the-counter medicines

As discussed in Chapter 2, these are products that are available to the public without a prescription (see 'Categories of medicines' on pp48–9). They include traditional pharmacy preparations and drugs that have more recently been deregulated from their previous status as prescription-only medicines (POMs) (one example of such a drug is Viagra), as well as herbal supplements, vitamins and mineral agents. The use of CAMs is increasing through patients' self-care with over-the-counter products (Cramer et al., 2010).

The UK government's patient choice agenda states a desire to support patients to make informed choices about their healthcare. CAMs are being sold in small specialist health shops, as well as pharmacies and supermarkets. Specialist health shops, pharmacies and supermarkets are all accessible to most individuals, and advice can be sought without delay.

Home remedies

Home remedies are made at home, are usually harmless when compared to other forms of modern medicines and rarely cause reactions or side effects. The popular belief with respect to home remedies is that they merely consist of consuming herbs, fruit juices and vegetable juices. The most common ingredients generally used in preparing these natural remedies include basil leaves, cardamom, cinnamon, fenugreek, onion, ginger, garlic, honey, pineapple, apple cider vinegar, turmeric, lemon, dandelion leaves, rose hips, horsetail, flaxseed, chamomile, olive oil, the outer leaves of cabbage, green tea, cranberry juice, orange juice, spinach juice and carrot juice. Home remedies come in many forms, including gargling a saline solution, drinking turmeric powder in milk, applying teabags, drinking herbal teas, applying cold or hot compresses, bath water, deodorants, mouth wash, nasal sprays, ear drops, liniments and poultices.

Home remedy protocols are required for liability purposes. If your patient in hospital asks to use a home remedy, you must ensure that there is a written instruction that has been drawn up and agreed in consultation with a doctor or pharmacist. The protocol should state the medicinal product that can be administered, indicating its use, the dose and the frequency (NMC, 2007b, 2008).

CAMs and home remedy interactions/contraindications with conventional medicines

Case study

Nigel, a staff nurse, was undertaking a morning drug round. He overheard a patient complaining about constipation to a healthcare assistant. The healthcare assistant suggested that the patient eat liquorice and low-sugar mints, as well as drinking plenty of fluids. Nigel approached the patient and healthcare assistant and explained that, prior to following this advice, the drug chart needed to be checked for possible drug interactions.

Interactions between drugs can be pharmacodynamic or pharmacokinetic in nature. Pharmacodynamic interactions occur when a drug inhibits the actions of another drug. Pharmacokinetic interactions occur as a result of a drug interfering with absorption, distribution, metabolism or excretion of another drug. The literature suggests that there are interactions between herbal medicines and conventional drugs. Examples of these are listed in Table 4.1 overleaf.

It is therefore extremely important that nurses are aware of the CAMs used by patients, and the interactions that occur between CAMs and conventional medicines. Nurses must take a thorough assessment of each patient to ascertain the medication (including CAMs, home remedies and conventional medications) that their patient is currently taking. They need to be competent in using the BNF. Having a good relationship, and the ability to converse with the pharmacist regarding potential drug interactions is pertinent in this process. If the nurse suspects a drug interaction, he or she must inform the patient, the pharmacist and the doctor, and provide written documentation in the patient's records. Medicines may be withheld according to the nurse's local Trust policy.

CAM	Interacts with
St John's wort	amitriptyline, ciclosporin, digoxin, erythromycin, midazolam, omeprazole, warfarin, loperamide
Ginkgo	omeprazole, anti-epileptics, aspirin, diuretics, ibuprofen, warfarin
Ginseng	warfarin
Garlic	chlorpropamide, warfarin
Echinacea	midazolam

Table 4.1: Interactions between herbal and conventional medicines

This section has focused on home remedies and over-the-counter remedies. It is important that you know about potential interactions between CAMs and prescribed medicines, and it is essential that you know the actions to take if you suspect interactions.

Nursing and CAMs

Holistic nursing care focuses on healing the whole person through the unity of body, mind, emotion, spirit and environment. Holistic nursing features a higher awareness of self, others, nature and spirit. Florence Nightingale had the same attitude, which focused on unity, wellness and the interrelationship of human beings, besides their environment. Holistic nurses may use CAMs. They incorporate people's physiological, psychological and spiritual needs into their care and believe that these enhance the healing process of clinical practices, rather than negate them.

Roles and responsibilities of the nurse in the administration of CAMs

While you have been introduced to some of the roles and responsibilities of the nurse in medicines administration in Chapter 2 (these will be covered in further detail in Chapter 5), it is pertinent that you are able to understand these roles and responsibilities in relation to CAMs.

The NMC (2008) recommends that nurses must support people to improve and maintain their own health, recognise and respect the contribution that people make to their own care and well-being, listen and respond to the concerns and preferences of their patients, and share information regarding the use of complementary or alternative therapies. Nurses have an obligation to respect the personal choices their patients make. Each nurse who wishes to practise a complementary or alternative therapy also has a responsibility to ensure that they have successfully undertaken training and are competent to practise. Nurses intending to incorporate CAMs into their nursing practice should only do so with the support, and in full knowledge, of their line manager, and in accordance with an established and agreed protocol.

Activity 4.9   *Critical thinking*

Revisit the case study at the beginning of this chapter. What NMC recommendations has the midwife failed to follow?

An outline answer is provided at the end of the chapter.

As you have learnt from Activity 4.9, a qualified nurse must work within the framework of the NMC *Code* (NMC, 2008) and the nurse in the case study does not appear to have done so.

Activity 4.10   *Communication*

Nurse Chen was working as a practice nurse at a GP surgery. During a consultation Jonas, a 69-year-old patient, admitted that he was feeling stressed and suffering from regular headaches. On further examination Nurse Chen found that Jonas was hypertensive. During the discussion the use of CAMs arose. Nurse Chen also practises aromatherapy. What information should Nurse Chen give to Jonas?

An outline answer is provided at the end of the chapter.

As you have learnt in Activities 4.9 and 4.10, it is essential for qualified nurses to be aware of their own prejudices and to share current, reliable research literature with their patients.

Assessment

Case study

Harold, 80 years old, was admitted to a medical ward. The admission process had been cut short due to an emergency on the ward. Eileen, the night nurse, was undertaking a drug round when she observed Harold taking a bottle of tablets out of his pocket. Eileen had been informed that Harold was not self-medicating. Eileen asked Harold to refrain from taking the tablets until she had completed his admission. During this assessment Eileen established that the medicine was a multivitamin and that this drug did not interact with any of the other medication Harold was taking. Harold was able to self-medicate this drug once it had been prescribed on his drug chart.

As you have learnt from the case study, assessment underpins the nursing care administered to the patient. A good assessment will include both current and historical information that focuses on biological, social and psychological functioning, as well as environmental and lifestyle factors that affect the individual's health. Information regarding current medicines (conventional and CAMs) is essential so that nurses can advise patients about drug interactions/contraindications.

During a visit to a pre-assessment clinic (prior to surgery for a right knee replacement), Doris reported that she was taking garlic. Garlic, as well as being antiseptic and antiviral, can thin the blood. What advice should the nurse give to Doris?

An outline answer is provided at the end of the chapter.

As you have learnt from Activity 4.11, taking garlic can thin the blood and bleeding may be prolonged. The nurse should advise Doris to stop taking this medication at least two weeks prior to her surgery.

This section has highlighted the importance of the role of nurses in medicines management and their responsibilities in this process. The importance of assessment, drug knowledge and communication with the pharmacist and patient has been highlighted, particularly in relation to drug interactions.

Health and safety of CAMs

If you assist with the administration of any form of CAM, it is important that you undertake the required infection control precautions. The National Institute for Clinical Excellence (NICE, 2003) has identified a number of standard principles that provide guidance on infection control precautions that should be applied by all healthcare personnel and carers. The recommendations are divided into three areas: hand hygiene, the use of personal protective equipment and the safe use and disposal of sharps. For example, you must always ensure that you wash or decontaminate your hands prior to administering a herbal remedy to a patient, or if a patient is receiving acupuncture, proper sharps disposal and decontamination of the equipment used is necessary.

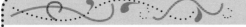

Chapter summary

This chapter has defined CAMs and explored their history. Arguments regarding their validity and efficacy have been addressed. We have learnt about the many different types of complementary and alternative therapies, their interactions and contraindications. Factors affecting patient choice were discussed. Nursing considerations were identified, namely professionalism and infection control. A more in-depth understanding of CAMs in your patient care will not only advance your knowledge but also increase patient safety and improve patient care.

Activities: brief outline answers

Activity 4.3 St John's wort and liquorice (page 96)

- Patients with bipolar disease or severe depression may experience mania if St John's wort is consumed. Patients with Alzheimer's disease and dementia should also avoid this herb because it can provoke psychotic delirium.
- Patients with chronic heart failure or hypertension should not use liquorice because of its mineralo-corticoid activity. Liquorice may cause hypertension or stimulate uterine contractions.

Activity 4.4 Herbal and prescribed medicine interactions (page 96)

There are numerous drug interactions, for example:

- ephedra should not be given with monoamine oxidase inhibitors;
- lily of the valley should not be prescribed in conjunction with digitalis as they could increase the power of each other.

Activity 4.5 Homeopathy (page 97)

Patients are instructed to avoid coffee, peppermint or menthol as these substances are thought to counteract the effect of the homeopathic remedy.

Activity 4.6 Insomnia, anxiety and CAMs (page 99)

A nurse must give the person asking for advice non-biased information about the CAMs to allow them to make an informed decision. There is a large number of CAMs used to treat insomnia (e.g. acupuncture, aromatherapy and therapeutic touch) and anxiety (e.g. therapeutic touch, distraction, relaxation and visualisation). Discuss these, including any contraindications, so that Sheila and James's mother can make informed choices.

Activity 4.8 Pain relief (page 104)

Discuss each of the CAMs that may help the patient's pain (e.g. acupuncture, aromatherapy, therapeutic touch, humour/laughter therapy, hypnosis, massage, meditation, distraction therapy, TENS, reflexology, relaxation, visualisation and reiki), including any contraindications, so that Reena can make an informed choice.

Activity 4.9 Midwife dismissive of CAMs (page 107)

The midwife in the case study does not appear to have:

- been non-judgemental about the patient's view;
- shared reliable information with the patient;
- been aware of current research literature;
- been aware of her own prejudices (for or against any particular CAM).

Activity 4.10 Relieving hypertension (page 107)

Discuss each of the CAMs that may relieve stress and the consequent hypertension (e.g. massage, aromatherapy, homeopathy and humour/laughter therapy), including any contraindications (without bias towards aromatherapy), so that Jonas can make an informed choice. The nurse must be aware of his or her own prejudices towards a given therapy.

Activity 4.11 Taking garlic (page 108)

The nurse should advise Doris to stop taking garlic two weeks before her admission for her knee replacement and should educate Doris about the benefits and contraindications of this plant.

Knowledge review

Now that you've worked through the chapter, how would you rate your knowledge of the following topics?

	Good	Adequate	Poor
1. The different types of alternative and complementary medicines.			
2. The factors that influence patient choice in medicines management.			
3. The health and safety aspects associated with the use of CAMs.			
4. The implications associated with the use of conventional medicines versus CAMs.			
5. The application of non-pharmacological methods to treat pain.			

Where you're not confident in your knowledge of a topic, what will you do next?

Further reading

Nursing and Midwifery Council (NMC) (2008) *The Code: Standards of conduct, performance and ethics for nurses and midwives* London NMC.

This document explains what is expected of nurses with regard to their professional conduct.

Peters, D (2008) *Family Guide to Complementary and Conventional Medicine.* London: Dorling Kindersley.

This is a readable book explaining the use of complementary, over-the-counter and conventional medicines.

Royal College of Nursing (RCN) (2003) *Complementary Therapies in Nursing, Midwifery and Health Visiting Practice.* London: RCN.

This book explores the use of many complementary therapies within nursing.

Useful websites

www.nmc-uk.org

You can access this website to read about the code of professional conduct and medicine management standards.

Chapter 5
Medicines administration

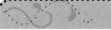

NMC Essential Skills Clusters

This chapter will address the following ESCs:

Cluster: Organisational aspects of care

20. People can trust the newly registered graduate nurse to select and manage medical devices safely.

By the first progression point:

1. Safely uses and disposes of medical devices under supervision and in keeping with local and national policy and understands reporting mechanisms relating to adverse incidents.

Cluster: Infection prevention and control

21. People can trust the newly registered graduate nurse to identify and take effective measures to prevent and control infection in accordance with local and national policy.

By the first progression point:

1. Follows local and national guidelines and adheres to standard infection control precautions.

22. People can trust the newly registered graduate nurse to maintain effective standard infection control precautions and apply and adapt these to needs and limitations in all environments.

By the first progression point:

1. Demonstrates effective hand hygiene and the appropriate use of standard infection control precautions when caring for all people.

25. People can trust a newly registered graduate nurse to safely apply the principles of asepsis when performing invasive procedures and be competent in aseptic technique in a variety of settings.

26. People can trust the newly qualified nurse to act, in a variety of environments including the home care setting, to reduce risk when handling waste, including sharps, contaminated linen and when dealing with spillages of blood and other body fluids.

Cluster: Medicines management

36. People can trust the newly registered graduate nurse to ensure safe and effective practice in medicines management through comprehensive knowledge of medicines, their actions, risks and benefits.

By the second progression point:

1. Uses knowledge of commonly administered medicines in order to act promptly in cases where side effects and adverse reactions occur.

37. People can trust the newly registered graduate nurse to safely order, receive, store and dispose of medicines (including controlled drugs) in any setting.

By the second progression point:

1. Demonstrates ability to safely store medicines under supervision.

... continued overleaf ...

continued . . .

38. People can trust the newly registered graduate nurse to administer medicines safely and in a timely manner, including controlled drugs.

By the second progression point:

1. Uses prescription charts correctly and maintains accurate records.
2. Utilises and safely disposes of equipment needed to draw up and administer medication, for example, needles, syringes, gloves.
3. Administers and, where necessary, prepares medication safely under direct supervision, including orally and by injection.

40. People can trust the newly registered graduate nurse to work in partnership with people receiving medical treatments and their carers.

By the second progression point:

1. Under supervision involves people and their carers in administration and self-administration of medicines.

Chapter aims

By the end of this chapter, you should be able to:

* understand the role of the nurse in the safe administration of medicines;
* identify the signs and symptoms of anaphylaxis and describe the care of a patient with anaphylaxis;
* understand the importance of adverse incident reporting;
* describe the concept of polypharmacy and how to minimise its adverse effects;
* understand the roles and responsibilities of the nurse in the self-administration of medicines;
* describe the key points for ordering, receiving, storing and disposing of medicines, including controlled drugs;
* understand the necessary infection control measures to take when preparing, dispensing and administering medicines.

Introduction

Case study

A woman was given misoprostol, a chemical abortion medication, after a nurse confused two patients, both with the same first name. Both women were attending a clinic that offers sterilisation, abortions and vasectomies. Patient A was attending for an initial consultation and Patient B was attending to have medication for the second stage of her medical abortion. To maintain patient confidentiality it was customary practice in the clinic to call out only the first name of each patient when invited to the consultation room. Once patients entered the private room, further checks, including full name, address and date of birth, were usually carried out. The nurse failed to do this when Patient A entered the room. Patient A was subsequently administered the medication that had been intended for Patient B. Had the nurse carried out the necessary identity checks, this mistake would never have occurred.

(Source: Seamark, 2008.)

Incidents like this are far too common in healthcare. The stories highlighted by the media are ones with tragic outcomes, but there are far more that don't make the headlines. The impact has far-reaching consequences not only for the patient but also for their relatives and the healthcare professionals involved. At best, in these situations, the patient suffers no lasting ill effects, although trust in the NHS and its employees is often irreparably damaged. In this particular case, once the nurse had realised her mistake, she readily owned up to it. The NMC placed a three-year caution on her record.

This chapter discusses the role of the nurse in the safe administration of medicines. Accurate patient identity checks are just one of many ways you can maintain safety. It is important that you understand a wide range of issues that can put patients at risk of the consequences of unsafe practice. For example, knowing your patient's presenting condition and underlying health and medical condition will ensure that you do not administer any medicines that are likely to exacerbate any health problems they may have. Understanding how medicines interact, their side effects and any special precautions you must take when administering them to your patient will assist in keeping your patient safe.

You must also know how to deal with complications that may arise, such as your patient experiencing a side effect or a severe allergic reaction to a medicine (**anaphylaxis**). In the event that a medicine error occurs, such as the one in the last case study, you should understand both your role and responsibility and those of the registered nurse in managing such a situation, such as **adverse incident reporting**. This chapter will also address infection control issues associated with the preparation and administration of medicines. **Polypharmacy** is another area of concern in medicines management, particularly when dealing with the older patient. What polypharmacy is and the detrimental effects associated with it shall be explored together with suggestions to minimise its negative impact on the patient. We shall also discuss the concept of the **self-administration** of medicines. Finally, the receiving, ordering, storage and safe disposal of medicines will be reviewed along with particular considerations regarding specific classes of medicines.

Patient safety

The safety of your patients should be paramount in all nursing activities that you undertake. Patients and their families and friends entrust their care to nurses, student nurses and all members of the healthcare team. The NMC reminds us that all care we provide to our patients must be based on the principles of safe practice. In order to maintain safety you need to have the underpinning knowledge of care you are about to deliver to your patient. It is important that, as a student nurse, you are aware not only of your capabilities, but of your limitations as well. Things are less likely to go wrong and patient safety is less likely to be compromised if you are aware of what you are able and not able to do. You must seek the necessary supervision and support from your mentor, other registered nurses and relevant members of the interprofessional team to ensure your practice is safe and effective. As a student nurse, the NMC (2007b) states that you *must never administer/supply medicinal products without direct supervision.*

In Chapter 1 we saw that the most serious medicine errors occurred during the administration stage of medicines management. In this section we will consider the steps to take to minimise mistakes occurring when we administer medicines to our patients. We will also explore what should be done in the event of a patient suffering an **anaphylactic reaction** to a medicine.

Activity 5.1   *Reflection*

Using your knowledge of the activities that occur during the administration stage of medicines management, outline the types of errors that may occur. It will also be useful to consider why these errors occur. You could provide your answer in a table with 'Error' in one column and 'Why?' in another.

An outline answer is provided at the end of the chapter.

The six 'Rs'

When administering medicines there are six rights (commonly referred to as 'Rs') that the nurse must consider to ensure that they are administered in a safe and effective manner. These are outlined in Table 5.1 overleaf.

Let us look at these rights in a bit more detail and consider the importance of adhering to them when administering medicines to patients.

The 'R'	Action to take
Right patient	Check the identity of patient against their wristband (or by other checks such as a photograph, confirmation of personal details) and the prescription chart.
Right medicine	Check that the medicine is suitable for the patient, the prescription can be read, and it matches the label on the medicine bottle.
Right dose	Check that the correct dose has been prescribed and then dispensed.
Right route	Check that the prescribed route of administration is correct and that the dose is administered by the correctly prescribed route.
Right time	Check that the medicine is prescribed for the correct time and frequency and that it is administered accordingly.
Right documentation	Check that the correct documentation has been used to record on the prescription chart that the medicine has been given or withheld.

Table 5.1: The six 'Rs' of medicines administration

Right patient

It is very important to ensure that any medicine prescribed is given to the correct patient. The case study at the beginning of this chapter shows how surprisingly easy it is to get this wrong. Name bands are often used so that the name, date of birth and individual patient or hospital number are matched against the details on the prescription chart. You can confirm the patient's identity by asking them their full name and date of birth. But don't rely on this method for confirming the patient's identity: some patients may be confused, have dementia, or be unable to speak English.

Some patients may not be able to tolerate wearing wristbands. For example, very small children may try to remove them or residents living in a nursing home may feel they are being labelled by being made to wear one. Clearly, a person living in their own home, who perhaps has visits from the district nurse to administer them their medication, would not be expected to wear such identification. In these situations it is still important to have a system that does not rely solely on verbal confirmation by the patient. These situations can easily be dealt with, for example, by having a photograph of the patient attached to the prescription chart and perhaps having two members of staff confirm the patient's identity against the photograph. Ensuring that prescription charts are kept by the patient's bedside and keeping patients' individual medicines in close proximity of their bedsides in locked medicine cabinets are other measures that can help to reduce medicine errors involving the wrong patient. You must also gain **informed consent** from your patient before any care you give to them; this includes medicines administration (please refer to Chapter 2, pp57–60).

Activity 5.2   *Communication*

Consider the barriers that may exist within your particular patient group in being able to confirm their identity.

An outline answer is provided at the end of the chapter.

Right medicine

Sometimes it can be difficult to tell exactly which medicine your patient has been prescribed, and this can be for a variety of reasons. Illegible handwriting by the prescriber may make the prescription difficult, if not impossible, to read. Any doubts arising from the legibility of the prescription must immediately be brought to the prescriber's attention. Using abbreviations instead of the full name of the medicine, either on the prescription chart or on the medicine packaging, may cause confusion. For example, the abbreviation 'MS' could mean morphine sulphate or magnesium sulphate. This is one reason why non-approved abbreviations should never be used in healthcare. Unfamiliarity with medicine names, medicines with similar names and similar packaging also compound the risk of giving the wrong medicine to your patient. It is vital that you read each medicine prescription carefully.

During a practical medicine administration examination a student nurse incorrectly verbalised a prescription as nitrazepam when in actual fact it read naproxen. The fictitious patient ended up receiving night sedation at 8 a.m. instead of their analgesia. Imagine if this had occurred in a real clinical setting.

Right dose

It is essential to be familiar with the usual dose range for the medicine prescribed; that way you will quickly recognise if a dose is unusual and may be incorrect. However, some medicines are used for more than one condition, and the normal dose ranges will be different. For example, carbamazepine is used to control epilepsy. In adult patients a dose of 400mg twice a day would be quite normal. This medicine can also be used for prophylaxis of bipolar disorder. For this condition, a dose of 200mg twice a day would be quite normal for an adult patient. Therefore, as well as being familiar with the usual dose of the medicines you are administering, you must know why your patient is taking the medicine. The preparation of a medicine may also determine its dose. For example, medicines dispensed in liquid form may require different doses to medicines dispensed in tablet form. One reason to explain why this is so is because liquids will be absorbed into the bloodstream a lot quicker than tablets. Therefore, they will act more quickly on the patient. It does not always correlate that the same dose of a medicine dispensed in one form will be the same for a medicine dispensed in a different form. A typical example is digoxin. Digoxin 125mcg dispensed in tablet form will be equivalent to digoxin 100mcg dispensed for intravenous use.

Some medicines and, in particular, those given to children are prescribed according to the weight or body surface area of the patient (see Chapter 1, pp35–7). Ensuring that you administer the correct dose to your patient requires you to have the necessary numeracy skills. As a student nurse you will always administer medicines under the direct supervision of a registered nurse, so do ensure that any medicine calculations are double-checked. Remember, if the dose you have calculated requires you to administer a large number of tablets or a fraction of a tablet, your calculation may be incorrect. Further problems that can lead to the wrong dose being administered can be further exacerbated by poor handwriting on the prescription chart. When checking the dose on the medicine packaging you must also ensure that you check that the medicine has not expired.

Right route

The medicine must always be given by the correct route to ensure that the pharmacodynamics of the medicine are not affected (you may wish to refer back to Chapter 3, pp81–3). It is important that you note the correct route as some medicines can only be administered via certain routes. As discussed, some doses of medicines may also need to be altered depending on the route of administration. Patients can become seriously ill or even die if a medicine is given by the wrong route.

Right time

It is important that the patient receives their medicine at the correct time. Some medicines are only meant to be given at specific times, for example night sedation. If zopiclone was administered to your patient at 8 a.m. instead of 10 p.m., think of the consequences for your patient: you may have a very drowsy patient to care for who may be at risk of a fall because of sleepiness. Other medicines need to be given at mealtimes with food, or before mealtimes and on an empty stomach, to enable them to work most effectively. Some medicine charts will have a section by each prescribed medicine where the prescriber or the pharmacist can include additional instructions or directions for how that medicine should be taken (for example, with food or swallowed whole). It is also necessary to ensure that some medicines are given at regular intervals throughout a 24-hour period. Antibiotics are an example of medicines that may be given four times a day. Administering antibiotics every six hours will ensure that therapeutic levels of the medicine are maintained in the bloodstream.

Right documentation

Medicine errors can also occur when documentation procedures are not thoroughly adhered to. For example, if a medicine is prescribed but not administered it should be documented on the prescription chart (and any other relevant pieces of documentation, as per Trust policy) to denote that it has not been given and the reason for this omission. Imagine you are confronted with a prescription chart inadequately completed by the previous nurse. If a signature box was left blank next to the time a medicine should have been given, you would not know why this was so. It could be because the medicine was not given and the nurse forgot to note this on the chart, or it could mean that the medicine was in fact administered but the nurse forgot to sign that the patient took it. Whatever subsequent action you take as a result could have consequences for your patient.

Activity 5.3 — *Decision-making*

It is 8 a.m. You have just received handover from the night staff and are now administering medicines, under the direct supervision of your mentor. You are at the bedside of Alice Sulah, a six-month-old baby admitted to the ward with a chest infection. You and your mentor are consulting her prescription chart and notice that her antibiotics, which were due for administration at 6 a.m., have not been signed for.

Consider the consequences for Alice if you choose to:

(a) administer the antibiotic that was due for 6 a.m.;
(b) not administer the antibiotic that was due for 6 a.m.

An outline answer is provided at the end of the chapter.

Knowledge of medical history

Another important consideration when administering medicines is your patient's presenting, underlying and previous medical conditions. This is because any medicines you administer to your patient may exacerbate or disguise a health problem. You must also be aware of any allergies your patient has, which includes food allergies. It is also best practice to ask your patient if they know of any intolerance they have to any medicines. For example, a patient may tell you that he or she feels nauseous when taking paracetamol. This does not necessarily mean the same as being allergic to paracetamol, but nevertheless is would be better to ask the doctor in this case to prescribe an alternative analgesic.

Contraindications, side effects and cautions when using medicines

You must have sound knowledge of any medicine you administer to your patients (including its pharmacodynamic and pharmacokinetic properties). Just because a medicine has been prescribed by a doctor, you should not automatically assume that it is safe or appropriate to administer. It is also necessary to familiarise yourself with the medicines you are administering to your patient to ensure that they should not be taken, where advised, with other medication. You should use the BNF if necessary. Therefore, before you administer any medicines to your patients, you must make sure that you are aware of any contraindications, side effects or special precautions that should be adhered to.

Maintaining accurate records

As you have learnt from Activity 5.3, if complete and accurate records are not maintained, you could be putting your patient at risk by committing a medicines management error. Most Trusts will have a recording system that you should use on the patient's prescription chart to denote whether a medicine has been administered to the patient or not. Figure 5.1 shows the front page of a typical prescription chart. You can see the codes that this particular organisation uses to indicate the reasons why medicines are not administered. Remember that, as a student nurse, any medicines you administer under the direct supervision of a registered nurse must be countersigned by them.

Controlled drugs (CDs) also require that accurate records are maintained when a patient is administered them. It is best practice that two nurses check the CD out from stock, record it in a controlled drugs record book and sign that the patient has taken that medicine.

The general rules of record keeping apply to the maintenance of medicine records, such as prescription charts. These rules include that any entry made on the prescription chart or in the controlled drugs record book should be in permanent ink; any errors made should be scored through with a single line, so that the error can still be read, and the amendment should be signed and dated; signatures or initials (where approved) should be legible and there should be a record kept on the ward of individual staff members' names, signatures and initials. You must sign for any medicine you have administered straightaway, in order to minimise the risk of a medicine error occurring (see Figure 5.2).

Valley Hills NHS Foundation Trust					

SURNAME	FORENAME	DATE OF BIRTH	PATIENT IDENTIFICATION NUMBER	ALLERGIES
HEIGHT	**WEIGHT**	**CONSULTANT**	**SPECIAL DIETARY REQUIREMENTS**	

ABBREVIATIONS

IV	Intravenous	1	Patient refused
IM	Intramuscular	2	Patient not on ward
S.C.	Subcutaneously	3	Not in stock
O	Orally	4	Contraindicated
S.L.	Sublinguinally		
TOP	Topically		
INH	Inhalation		
PR	Per rectum		

ONCE ONLY DRUGS/VARIABLE DOSE PRESCRIPTIONS

Date	Drug	Dose	Route	Prescriber's signature	Administered by	Date and time	Pharmacy

Figure 5.1: A typical prescription chart

SURNAME Bridges	FORENAME Beryl	DATE OF BIRTH 01/11/1930	PATIENT IDENTIFICATION NUMBER 143986	ALLERGIES None known
HEIGHT 1.65m	**WEIGHT** 65kg	**CONSULTANT** Langley	**SPECIAL DIETARY REQUIREMENTS** None	

ONCE ONLY DRUGS/VARIABLE DOSE PRESCRIPTIONS

Date	Drug	Dose	Route	Prescriber's signature	Administered by	Date and time	Pharmacy
29/09/10	Clexane	20mg	S.C	R. Wright	M. Arkah	29/09/10 at 06.00	

REGULAR PRESCRIPTIONS

				Time	Date									
Drug Digoxin				08.00										
Route 0	Dose 125mcg	Start Date 29/09/10	End Date 03/10/10											
Prescriber's Signature R. Wright		Pharmacy												
Drug Lactulose				08.00										
Route 0	Dose 10ml	Start Date 29/09/10	End Date 03/10/10											
Prescriber's Signature R. Wright		Pharmacy		20.00										
Drug Amoxicillin				06.00										
Route I.V	Dose 500mg	Start Date 29/09/10	End Date 03/10/10	14.00										
Prescriber's Signature R. Wright		Pharmacy		22.00										
Drug Paracetamol				06.00										
Route P.R	Dose 1g	Start Date 29/09/10	End Date 03/10/10	12.00 18.00										
Prescriber's Signature R. Wright		Pharmacy		24.00										

Figure 5.2: A completed prescription chart

Your hospital may use electronic prescription charts. If this is the case, there will be a policy for recording electronically any medicines administered or omitted. The policy will also detail how any errors made should be electronically recorded so that, where necessary, they can be traced back to the individual concerned.

Knowing how to read and interpret your individual hospital Trust's prescription chart is vital to ensure that you dispense and administer the correct medicine to the right patient. Accurate documentation is extremely important and serves as a permanent record of a particular nursing intervention you gave to your patient at a specified point in time.

Anaphylaxis

This section will discuss the potentially fatal condition of anaphylaxis. While there is much you can do to ensure safety in medicines management, on rare occasions you may be faced with providing emergency care to a patient who has suffered anaphylaxis as a result of a medicine he or she has been given. Consider the following true story.

Case study

Teresa Innes, a 38-year-old mother, suffered anaphylaxis after being given penicillin to treat an abscess on her leg. She had recently returned from a holiday to Corfu, where she sustained an insect bite. It became infected and on her return home to the UK she was prescribed a non-penicillin antibiotic by her GP. After a week there was no improvement and she was referred to hospital for a minor operation to treat a leg abscess. In preparation for the operation a hospital doctor prescribed penicillin, despite her medical notes and wristband clearly indicating her allergy. Post-mortem results showed that she had suffered brain damage due to lack of oxygen caused by an anaphylactic reaction to penicillin.

This tragic story could have been avoided had the healthcare practitioners responsible for Teresa's care taken note of her penicillin allergy.

Anaphylaxis is a medical emergency. It is a severe allergic reaction to something and has the potential to be fatal. It occurs when an **allergen** is introduced either on to or into the body for the second time. In the case of a medicine being an allergen, the patient will have initially been exposed to it on a previous occasion. The body produces **antibodies** against the medicine. When the same medicine is introduced to the body again, the antibodies react with specific cells called **mast cells** to bring about a sudden release of chemical substances, including histamine, into the bloodstream and surrounding tissues. The most commonly implicated medicines are antibiotics, anaesthetic medicines and NSAIDs. The Resuscitation Council (UK) (2008) offers very useful guidelines on how to recognise and deal with incidences of anaphylaxis.

Signs and symptoms of anaphylaxis

Patients can suddenly become very unwell. The speed with which anaphylaxis happens is dependent on the route the allergen entered the body. In the case of the allergen being a medicine, it will happen more quickly if the medicine is given directly into the bloodstream via the intravenous route. Symptoms usually present within 3 to 60 minutes of the allergen being introduced into the patient's body. Usually life-threatening airway, breathing and/or circulation problems occur. This can be accompanied by changes to the skin such as flushing, redness, itching or swelling. Patients can also experience gastrointestinal disturbances such as abdominal cramps or vomiting. They may also experience a sense of 'impending doom' and appear very anxious.

The airway can be affected by swelling of the throat or tongue. The patient may experience difficulty in swallowing as the airway narrows, and may have a **stridor**, which is characterised by noisy, high-pitched breathing or wheezing as air is being forced through the upper airway obstruction.

Breathing may become laboured and increase in rate. The patient may also become cyanosed (with pale or blue-tinged fingers and lips) as the oxygen levels in the blood diminish. After a short period of time the patient will become tired because of the increased effort required to breathe. He or she may also become confused due to **hypoxia**. If the condition is left untreated the patient may stop breathing.

Circulatory problems are characterised by an increased heart rate and decreased blood pressure. The patient may display typical signs of shock such as cool, pale, clammy skin, and may complain of feeling dizzy and lose consciousness. If left untreated the patient may go into cardiac arrest.

It is important to note that anaphylaxis is different from a severe allergic reaction. With a severe allergic reaction, patients may experience some of the symptoms listed above, but these will not include the life-threatening airway, breathing or circulation problems. The treatment for an allergic reaction will differ from that used to treat anaphylaxis.

Treatment of anaphylaxis

The outcome for the patient with anaphylaxis will very much depend on how quickly he or she is treated. If the patient is able to sit up (and is not **hypotensive**), this is preferable as it will make breathing easier for them. However, if the patient complains of feeling dizzy or faint, he or she should be assisted to lie down, as sitting or standing will further lower the blood pressure and may induce a cardiac arrest. Depending on the route of the administered allergen (in this case the medicine), it may be possible to stop the medicine from being administered. For example, if the patient was receiving the medicine intravenously, it may be possible to stop it. The Resuscitation Council (UK) (2008) advises that **adrenaline** should be administered as soon as possible. In a hospital situation, where there are experienced specialists to do so, this may be administered via the intravenous route for rapid onset of action. However, adrenaline must be given promptly, so in cases where there are not experienced specialists in the use of IV adrenaline, the intramuscular route should be used. In a community setting, for example, the healthcare professional would use the intramuscular route. The dose administered will be dependent on the age of the individual patient. The patient is also subjected to a **fluid challenge** whereby fluid is rapidly infused into the patient. The patient may have lost a large volume of fluid from his or her circulation during anaphylaxis. Antihistamines, steroids and oxygen therapy are also administered to the patient. Other medicines that may also be of use, depending on the signs and symptoms the patient is experiencing, are bronchodilators and certain cardiac medicines.

Any incidents of medicine-related anaphylaxis should also be reported to the Medicines and Healthcare products Regulatory Agency (MHRA). The 'Yellow Card' reporting system is in place whereby a healthcare professional completes a Yellow Card when they suspect a patient has had an adverse reaction to medicine. These cards can be found at the back of a BNF or can be completed on line at **www.yellowcard.gov.uk**.

Adverse incident reporting

As you can see from the sections above, there is much that you can do to keep your patients safe when administering medicines. Inevitably, mistakes will happen, despite your best efforts to maintain safe practice. Statistics tell us that often mistakes are not just random events and that they usually occur as a result of weaknesses in the NHS, such as flawed policies, poor resources or overworked staff. However, what is important is that we learn from such mistakes and put measures in place in an attempt to ensure that they do not happen again. It is therefore essential that, when mistakes happen, they are reported straightaway, primarily to ensure that no harm is caused to the patient, visitor or member of staff involved, but also to determine how the mistake happened in an effort to put systems in place to prevent such errors in the future. The important thing to remember when reporting mistakes is that it is the action taken as a result of that report that will determine whether that same mistake happens again. Reporting is just the first stage in the process of incident prevention.

Adverse incident reporting forms part of **clinical governance**, a system used in the NHS in which appropriate individuals are accountable for improving the quality and safeguarding the standards of care given to patients. The NHS has a 'no blame culture' to encourage staff to own up to mistakes so as to try to prevent them happening again. However, a completely blame-free culture is not appropriate for incidences where individuals make very serious mistakes due to sheer negligence or incompetence; then, it is only right that they are held to account.

What is an adverse incident?

Any errors that occur during the provision of healthcare can be termed adverse incidents. Other terms that you may hear are untoward events, **actual harm incidents** or **near-miss incidents** or events. Any processes involved in medicines management where mistakes are made have the potential to cause serious harm to your patients. These incidents are classified into 'actual harm' and 'near miss' incidents. Any omissions in patient care, such as forgetting to give a patient their medicine, or not remembering to sign the prescription chart for a medicine administered, are also classified as adverse incidents. Regardless of whether the patient was harmed, all incidents should be reported and documented. You will need to refer to your particular hospital Trust policy regarding the steps that should be taken when reporting incidents.

Near-miss incidents

A near-miss incident can be described as an unexpected occurrence that did not result in any harm (be that physical or psychological) to the patient. This is because the incident was prevented from happening. The Department of Health (DH, 2000) has described it as:

a situation in which an event or omission, or a sequence of events or omissions, arising during clinical care fails to develop further, whether or not as a result of compensating action, thus preventing injury to a patient.

Actual harm incidents

Incidents that were not prevented from happening, and that result in harm or have the potential to cause harm in any way, are described as actual harm incidents. The Department of Health (DH, 2000) offers their definition:

an adverse health care event (AHCE) is an event or omission arising during clinical care and causing physical or psychological injury to a patient.

How are incidents reported?

It is important that incidents are reported as soon as possible after they have happened. This is to ensure that any harm that may have been caused to your patient as a result of the incident is minimised as much as possible. Another reason why it is so important to report it immediately is so that it can be investigated promptly and measures put in place to prevent a similar incident from happening again.

Your hospital Trust will have its own incident reporting policy. Should you be involved in or witness an adverse incident, you will be expected to report it. Your Trust will expect you to complete an incident report form either in writing or electronically. Figure 5.3 outlines the type of information that should be completed on an incident report form. Please note that this is a very much simplified version of an incident form. In practice your forms may be longer and in some Trusts you will be expected to input records of adverse incidents into a computer. The incident describes a patient who was administered the wrong dose of a medicine.

Activity 5.4 *Critical thinking*

Look at the incident form in Figure 5.3 overleaf.

(a) Was this an actual harm or a near-miss incident?
(b) Summarise in your own words, in one sentence, what actually happened in this incident.

An outline answer is provided at the end of the chapter.

While most medicine management errors can be avoided, this section has enabled you to realise the importance of reporting such errors to minimise their impact on the patient and to reduce their prevalence in the future.

SURNAME	FORENAME	GENDER	DATE OF BIRTH	PATIENT IDENTIFICATION NUMBER
Sullivan	Bridget	Male Female ✓	18/10/34	9630369

DEPARTMENT WARD	EXACT LOCATION OF THE INCIDENT	DATE OF INCIDENT
Ash Ward	Bay A Bed 3	9/3/10 **TIME OF INCIDENT** 18.05

CATEGORY (please tick)

In-patient   Visitor
Out-patient ✓   Employee

PLEASE PROVIDE AN ACCURATE DESCRIPTION OF THE INCIDENT (continued overleaf if necessary)

It was 18.05 and I was administering the 18.00 hours medicines to Mrs Bridget Sullivan on 9th March 2010. The prescription chart read to administer 30mg of dihydrocodeine via the oral route at 18.00 hours. In error I dispensed three tablets of 15 mg (45mg in total) into the medicine pot and then administered the tablets to Mrs Sullivan. I realised my error as soon as Mrs Sullivan had swallowed the tablets. I immediately informed Mrs Sullivan of my mistake, explaining to her that I should have administered her two tablets of 15mg instead of 3 tablets of 15 mg. I performed a set of clinical observations on Mrs. Sullivan. These were within normal parameters (see observations recorded in box below). I informed the nurse in charge of my mistake, Sr Joan Bilboe at 18.10. I also informed Dr. Morris of the error at 18.15. Mrs Sullivan was commenced on 15 minute observations for 2 hours.

TYPE OF INCIDENT (e.g. Fall, Medication error, Equipment failure)	OBSERVATIONS	WHAT WAS THE INJURY? (e.g. lacerations, bruise, fracture, unconsciousness, etc.)
Medication error	Blood pressure: 130/85mmHg Temperature: 36.8° C Pulse: 78 b.p.m Respiration: 16 r.p.m	No apparent injury

TREATMENT GIVEN/ACTION TAKEN	NAME OF WITNESS(ES) TO INCIDENT:
Clinical observations taken and recorded. Patient commenced on 15 minute observations for 2 hours	Gail Decoats

MEMBER OF STAFF INCIDENT REPORTED TO:	CONTACT DETAILS OF WITNESSES
Sr Joan Bilboe and Dr Morris	Gail Decoats Ash Ward Tel: 0123 4567

I CONFIRM THESE DETAILS ARE AN ACCURATE ACCOUNT OF THE INCIDENT

Signed: Gail Decoats   Date: 9/3/10   **Designation:** Staff Nurse

Figure 5.3: A simplified incident report form

Infection control in medicines administration

Preventing and controlling the spread of infection is one of the most important roles you will undertake. It underpins practically all aspects of nursing care. In this section we will look at specific infection control measures to take when preparing and administering medicines, which have been briefly covered in Chapter 4.

When preparing medicines for administration a **clean technique** is used. This means that your hands should be visibly clean. Depending on the medicine you are preparing, the route that it is going to be administered and the patient who will be receiving the medicine will determine whether you should wear **personal protective equipment (PPE)**. This may include all or some of the following: gloves, aprons, masks, visors, goggles, gowns or overshoes. The general principle remains the same for all medicines you are preparing for administration, which is that a clean, no-touch technique is used at all times. Your bare hands should never come into contact with a medicine you are going to administer to your patient. Apart from for infection control reasons, you may be allergic to the medicine or it may cause a skin reaction. When preparing injections an aseptic technique is used to ensure that all the equipment you use (syringes, needles and medicines) is kept sterile to reduce the risk of micro-organisms being introduced into the patient's body. Detailed below are the particular infection control precautions you should take when preparing and administering medicines via the various routes.

Intravenous, intramuscular and subcutaneous administration

When preparing medicines, where their route of entry will bypass the body's natural defences or when handling intravenous cannulae, an aseptic technique should be used to prevent any contamination of syringes, needles or cannulae. If your patient is receiving IV medicines, the nurse who is administering them must clean the injection port on the cannulae with an alcohol swab to reduce the risk of bacterial contamination. There is much debate over whether the patient's skin requires cleansing before the administration of a subcutaneous or intramuscular injection. Alcohol swabs are sometimes used to decontaminate the skin. The alcohol must be allowed to dry on the skin for about 30 seconds before administration of the injection; otherwise, the skin preparation is ineffective. The argument for not cleansing the skin before an injection is that the majority of a patient's skin is 'socially clean' and, as the nurse prepares the injection under strict hand hygiene and aseptic conditions, it is unlikely that micro-organisms would be introduced into the skin. There is also a risk that the use of alcohol will cause slight hardening of the skin. You will need to check what your hospital Trust's policy is regarding skin preparation and ensure that you adhere to it.

For all injections, regardless of their route, you must ensure that you perform thorough hand-washing and/or hand decontamination before preparing the injection. You may also need to wear PPE; this will depend on Trust policy, the medicines you are preparing and whether your patient is being **barrier nursed** for infection control reasons.

You must also remember to dispose of any sharp instruments you have used into an approved sharps bin. Another very important point to remember is that any needles that have been injected into the patient's skin (used needles) must never be re-sheathed. This is to reduce the risk of piercing your skin with a needle that is potentially contaminated with blood-borne viruses such as HIV or hepatitis B and C.

Intravesical, rectal and vaginal routes

With these routes, because you will be coming into contact with bodily fluids, you will need to wear PPE when administering medicines to your patient. As a minimum this will include gloves and aprons. You will also need to consider wearing gowns, masks, goggles or visors if there is a risk that you may become splashed with blood, bodily fluids or droplets from the medicine that is being administered. Depending on the medicine the patient is going to receive via these routes, it may also be necessary to wear gloves, aprons and even face visors when preparing the medicines for administration. For example, your patient may be receiving cytotoxic medicines via the intravesical route, which would be an irritant if it came into contact with your skin or eyes.

Transdermal or topical route

Medicine preparations administered transdermally may be dispensed in a patch format that is applied directly to the skin or in a cream or ointment that is rubbed into the skin. Once you have decontaminated your hands, you must wear disposable gloves prior to administering these medicines. This is to reduce the risk of introducing micro-organisms from your hands on to the patient's skin, and will prevent any of the medicine getting on to your skin. Always ensure that, after you remove your gloves, you wash your hands thoroughly, just in case any of the ointment has been transferred to your skin when you removed your gloves.

Oral, sublingual and buccal routes

It is not usual practice to wear gloves and aprons when dispensing or administering medicines via these routes. However, you must decontaminate your hands before the procedure. When dispensing the medicines make sure your hands do not come into contact with the tablet, capsule or liquid. When dispensing tablets or capsules from a bottle, tip it out into the bottle cap first; when you are sure you have dispensed the correct number of tablets or capsules, you can then transfer them into the medicine pot. The reason for this is that you do not touch the medicine and, if you tip too many tablets out into the cap, it is far easier to tip the excess tablets back into the bottle from the cap, rather than from the medicine pot, where you may have already dispensed other medicines. When dispensing tablets from blister packs, you should push the tablets from the back of the packaging through to the front. Do not peel the packaging away to expose the tablet as there is a risk that you will touch it with your hands. If your patient is unable to take the medicines from the pot, you should don disposable gloves to assist the patient. This will ensure your hands do not come into contact with the medicine or the patient's oral mucous membranes.

Nasal, inhalation, aural and ocular routes

Ointments and drops may become contaminated with micro-organisms as they are applied to your patient. Therefore, it is important that you observe their relatively short shelf life. Most of these medicines should be discarded seven days after opening. Once you have decontaminated your hands you should consider whether it is appropriate to wear gloves. For example, when administering eye drops or ointments you will need to gently pull down the lower eyelid to apply the medicine to the **conjunctival sac**. This may lead to your hands becoming contaminated with the medicine or fluid from the eye. Clean tissues or sterile swabs (depending on your hospital Trust policy) should be used to remove excess drops that may leak from the patient's eye. A separate tissue or swab should be used for each eye to prevent cross-contamination.

This section has highlighted the necessary precautions you should take when preparing and administering medicines to your patient in order to reduce the risk of spreading infection to either you or your patients.

Polypharmacy

Another area that needs to be considered in medicines management is polypharmacy. This section will explore what it means, its impact on the patient and what you can do to minimise its harmful effects. The term polypharmacy means taking several medicines ('poly' means many and 'pharmacy' refers to medicines) and is usually applied to a patient who takes more than four medicines at a time. It is more common among older adults.

Problems associated with polypharmacy

Polypharmacy has been implicated in a range of health concerns, particularly among older people, who are more likely to take a variety of different medicines for a range of medical conditions. Medicine-related problems are more likely to occur if someone is taking four or more medicines, has recently been discharged from hospital or is taking medicines such as warfarin, digoxin, diuretics or NSAIDs (DH, 2001b). Problems are further compounded when there becomes a blurring as to whether new medicines are being prescribed to treat a new medical condition or side effects associated with medicines already being taken by the patient.

Physiological changes attributed to ageing

To understand the problems that older people in particular may experience as a result of taking multiple medicines, you may need to refer back to Chapter 3 (pp69–70) to remind yourself of the principles of pharmacology. Older patients are at an increased risk of adverse reactions to their medicines. The processes involved in pharmacokinetics are thought to become slower with increasing age. For example, the acidity level in the stomach increases, which will alter the absorption rate of some medicines that require a less acidic environment to start being absorbed from the stomach into the bloodstream. The surface area of the bowel, which also plays a major role in the absorption process, is thought to decrease with age. This may have an impact on certain medicines, such as slow-release formulas. Changes in the body attributed to ageing may also affect the pharmacokinetic and pharmacodynamic processes involved in medicine therapy. Older people have reduced proportions of water in their body, which will result in much higher levels of water-soluble medicines, such as digoxin and gentamycin, in the bloodstream. The proportion of body fat increases with age and this will result in an increased half-life of medicines. Therefore **lipid soluble** medicines will stay in the bloodstream for longer. Examples of these medicines include diazepam. The liver is the main organ responsible for the metabolism of medicines. With increasing age the liver decreases in size, and blood flow and enzymatic activity decreases. The kidney is the main organ involved in the excretion of medicines from the body. Again, with the ageing process it loses mass, resulting in a decrease in the **glomerular filtration rate**, so medicines take longer to be excreted. The clearance rate can be further slowed down by conditions such as dehydration, reduced cardiac function and kidney disease.

Hospital admission and readmission

Polypharmacy may also be responsible for older patients being admitted to hospital – 5–17 per cent of unplanned hospital admissions are due to patients experiencing adverse reactions to their medicines. It is also thought that up to 50 per cent of older patients may not be taking their medicines as intended and, with 80 per cent of older adults in our society taking more than one medicine, this has the potential to cause a lot of problems (DH, 2001b).

Concordance with medicines regime

Polypharmacy has been associated with patients not taking their medicines as they should. The reasons why they may not comply with their medicines regime are as follows.

- They do not realise the importance of continuing with their medicines regime.
- Unpleasant side effects may be experienced with some medicines.
- Patients do not understand how and when their medicines should be taken; or patients may assume that they no longer require their medicines because their symptoms improve.
- Similar packaging may also cause confusion and for some patients, particularly those with manual dexterity problems, opening up medicines may be difficult.
- Patients may also choose not to take their medicines because the taste is unpalatable.
- They may be taking over-the-counter or herbal medicines that may result in them not taking their prescribed medicine, or it may be contraindicated.
- It may not be convenient for patients to take their medicines at the prescribed times.

Activity 5.5   *Critical thinking and decision-making*

Jacob Stein is a 93-year-old man who was admitted to your ward one week ago with dehydration and confusion. Prior to this admission, he was discharged from the surgical ward after undergoing a hernia repair. He also has a history of diabetes and osteoarthritis. He takes his 8 a.m. medicines in the morning in his bay, but at lunchtime in the dayroom he always declines, although the medicines are the same as in the morning. His prescribed medicines are as follows: diclofenac 50mg orally, three times daily; paracetamol 1g orally,

continued overleaf . . .

continued . . . .

four times daily; gaviscon 10ml orally, four times daily; metformin 500mg orally, three times daily, and nitrazepam 5mg orally, once daily at night time. When asked repeatedly to take his medications he declines, saying it is doing him no good and claiming that he is being poisoned by the staff.

(a) What reasons do you think are behind Jacob refusing his lunchtime medicines?
(b) What could you do to ensure that Jacob complies with his medicines regime?

An outline answer is provided at the end of the chapter.

Solutions to problems

The problems associated with polypharmacy are immense. It is therefore essential that care is planned and delivered in a holistic manner to ensure that the detrimental effects of polypharmacy are reduced.

Prescribing

When prescribing new medicines for patients their medical condition/s and current medicines should be taken into account. Prescribing should involve a multidisciplinary approach. Patients may be under the care of several different specialists who may all work independently of each other. It is important that all specialists involved in the patients' care only prescribe with full knowledge of all their medical conditions and prescribed medicines. Any over-the-counter or herbal remedies taken by the patient should also be noted and considered when reviewing the medicine regime. Some herbal remedies will have an effect on prescribed medicines. For example, St John's wort, used as a herbal remedy for mild to moderate depression, should not be taken with several kinds of medicine, including anticonvulsants, warfarin and digoxin. It is also recommended that patients over 75 years of age should have their medicines reviewed as part of a yearly health check-up. This should increase to every six months for patients taking four or more medicines. Blood tests should also be performed during these reviews to check that medicines are within therapeutic range in the patient's circulatory system.

Dispensing

Consideration to any manual dexterity or reading difficulties your patient may have should also be given when deciding how their medicines should be packaged. For example, many medicines dispensed in bottles have childproof caps designed to make them very difficult for a child to open. This can pose problems for your patient if he or she has poor hand grip or arthritic wrists or fingers. Large-print labels and instructions should be provided for those with visual impairment. If your patient has swallowing problems, you should liaise with the pharmacist to see if any of their medicines can be dispensed in liquid form or dispersible tablets. Some patients may also have their medicines dispensed in a **dosset box** (see Figure 5.4 overleaf). This is particularly useful for those patients who may have difficulties in remembering the exact times they should

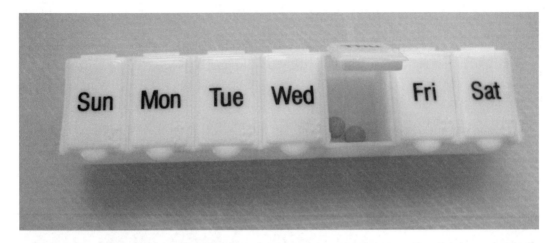

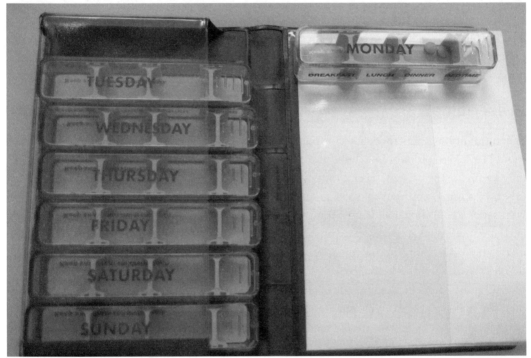

Figure 5.4: Two types of dosset box

take their medicines, cannot open bottle caps or boxed tablets easily, may be poorly sighted or may have difficulty reading the labels on the boxes or bottles. The patient's medicines are placed into the relevant compartments for the days of the week and the times they should be taken. Written instructions detailing exactly what the medicines are and their dose are also provided with the dosset box.

Administering

Patients need to be educated about the purpose, side effects, contraindications, particular precautions, dose, frequency and duration of their medicines to ensure **concordance** with the regime. It will also be useful to educate their carers if they are responsible for administering medicines to patients.

There is a lot you can do to ensure your patients are prescribed the correct medicines. Recognising the potential problems associated with polypharmacy will enable you to put a few simple measures in place to reduce the potential harmful impact on your patients.

Self-administration of medicines in hospitals

Self-administration of medicines enables a patient to have total or partial control over when they take their medicines. It is thought that, by allowing and encouraging this, clinical settings will improve the concordance rate among patients taking their medicines. As discussed earlier in this chapter, there is evidence to suggest that some patients do not take their medicines as intended, particularly older patients and those taking multiple medicines. By giving patients the responsibility to take their medicines, it is hoped that this will improve. In the case of children, the control over self-administration of medicines could be given to parents or carers. In this situation the parents or carers would need to have their ability assessed.

Medicine lockers

In order to facilitate the process, your patient will have an individual lockable storage area near the bed where their medicines will be kept. Medicines are then easily available when your patient needs to take them. Depending on your patient's cognitive and physical ability, he or she will be given their own key to the medicine locker, with a master key held by the registered nurse.

Patient assessment

Careful consideration must be given to determine whether your patient is able to self-administer medicines. A thorough assessment should be carried out to identify whether your patient is able to take full or partial control over when to take his or her medicines. The NMC (2007b) recommends that patients should be assessed on three levels for their suitability for self-administration.

- Level 1: the nurse remains responsible for the storage and administration of the medicine to the patient.
- Level 2: the nurse is responsible for the safe storage of the medicines. Patients ask the nurse to open their medicine lockers when their medicines are due and the nurse allows the patients to take their medicines out of the packaging and administer them under their direct supervision.
- Level 3: patients are totally independent at self-administration. They will need to prove that they know what medicines they are taking, why they are taking them, how they should be taken and when they are due. They will also need to prove that they have no cognitive deficits and have the manual dexterity to open the locked cupboard and take their medicines from the container that they are stored in. These patients will be given their own locker key and

have total control over when they take their medicines. The nurse will reassess the patients' ability on a regular basis, particularly as and when their conditions change. It must be remembered that the registered nurse is still accountable for patients taking their medicines.

Activity 5.6   *Critical thinking*

Consider the following patient scenarios.

(a) Priya Patel is a 48-year-old lady admitted to the ward for a mastectomy for breast cancer. She has no known previous medical history and is on the theatre list for tomorrow morning.
(b) Priya Patel (as above) has just returned to the ward following her mastectomy.
(c) Moira O'Regan is the mother of seven-year-old Teigan Bronte. Teigan Bronte has been admitted to the ward with a chest infection. Teigan also has Down's syndrome.
(d) Harrison Blakemore is 85 years old. He is poorly sighted and suffers with short-term memory loss.
(e) Derek Swinton is 32 years old. He is undergoing treatment for alcohol misuse. He also has a past history of drug misuse.

Decide whether each patient or carer should be allowed to self-administer their medicines and at what level (1, 2 or 3). Explain the reasons for your choices.

An outline answer is provided at the end of the chapter.

Ordering, receiving, storage and disposal of medicines

Another important aspect of medicines management you will need to know is how to order, receive, store and dispose of medicines safely and in line with your Trust policies. In clinical settings all medicines are controlled by the legislation outlined in Chapter 2. Particular legislation, such as the Medicines Act 1968, states how medicines should be labelled and the types of containers they should be stored in (HMSO, 1968). The Misuse of Drugs Act 1971 deals with controlled drugs (CDs) and their classes, and outlines the requirements that must be adhered to for the supply, possession, storage and destruction of CDs (HMSO, 1971). The Misuse of Drugs Regulations 2001 provide specific requirements on how controlled drugs should be supplied, stored and prescribed. They also deal with record keeping for controlled drugs (HMSO, 1973/2001).

Ordering medicines

It is best practice to ensure that stocks of medicines are kept at an adequate level in the area in which they are being used; this could be in a ward setting, in the pharmacy department or even in the patient's home. This will minimise the risk of the stock running out and there then being a delay in administering the medicine to your patient. Each Trust will have its own policy on the ordering of medicines. The general principles are that medicines are usually ordered by a registered nurse or the pharmacist. A stock order is completed, either on paper or online, and the order is sent to the pharmacy department for processing and dispensing. Individual wards and departments tend to have a list of the most commonly used medicines together with a desired stock level. It is usually the responsibility of the pharmacist to check the stock levels regularly (this may be every few days or weekly) and reorder any stocks of medicines that are running low.

Ordering controlled drugs

There are special considerations and restrictions imposed on ordering CDs, because they can be open to misuse and abuse. Hospital wards and departments usually hold a small stock of CDs. To order them the nurse has to complete a CD order form, which is in duplicate. This form requires the signature of an authorised nurse on the ward or department. These order forms must be stored in a locked cupboard when they are not being used. Records of ordering and administering CDs must be kept for two years.

Receiving medicines

Medicine stocks are usually brought to the ward for the registered nurse to check and then stored securely. The stocks should be checked against the order form by a registered nurse to ensure the correct medicines, doses and quantities have been received.

Receiving controlled drugs

CDs are taken to the clinical area in a sealed package. They must be accepted on to the ward by a registered nurse. Two registered nurses check the medicines against the order form, including the doses, expiry dates and number or volume of the tablets or ampoules. These are then added to the stock in the CD record book.

Storing medicines

The safe storage of medicines in a ward or department is the responsibility of the registered nurse in charge. Cupboards used for the storage of medicines must conform to the British Standard for Medicines Storage (BS2881). In the community, patients are advised to store their medicines in a safe place, away from the reach of children. They should also be reminded to read the information leaflets that accompany their medicines in order to find out in what type of conditions they should be stored. Storing medicines correctly will ensure that their active properties are not compromised and that only authorised individuals have access to them. It is the nurse in charge of the ward or department who has responsibility to ensure that all medicines are stored safely and securely. The nurse in charge is also responsible for controlling access to cupboards where medicines are stored. While in practical terms medicine keys are normally handed to other qualified nurses on duty throughout a shift, the responsibility remains with the nurse in charge. As a student nurse you should never hold the keys. All medicines should be stored in a locked cupboard or fridge (if appropriate) to ensure that there is no unauthorised access to them.

Medicines must also be stored in conditions that do not subject them to vast variations in temperature; for example, they should not be stored in direct sunlight or by radiators. You will need to look on a medicine's packaging to tell you within what temperature range that particular medicine can be safely stored. Generally, they should be stored in dry conditions where moisture is unlikely to seep into the packaging. Medicines should also be stored in the containers in which they have been dispensed by the pharmacy department. This is to ensure that instructions or any particular cautions are kept with the medicine. Some medicines are also stored in dark containers to minimise sunlight or daylight affecting their medicinal properties. It is also important to rotate stock: first in, first out. Placing items that will reach their expiry date sooner at the front of a medicine storage cupboard will ensure that you do not have piles of expired stock.

Storage of controlled drugs

The Misuse of Drugs (Safe Custody) Regulations 1973/2007 deal with the safe storage of CDs (HMSO, 1973/2007). To ensure they are safely stored, CDs should be kept in a specific locked cupboard within a second locked cupboard. Keys should only be made available to those with authorised access. For additional security there is a light situated on the outside of the cupboard to make it clearly visible to all staff when the cupboard is open or if it has not been locked. No other medicines should be stored in the CD cupboard. A regular stock check is made of CDs; this may be every 24 hours, according to local Trust policy.

Disposal of medicines

Medicines must be disposed of in accordance with legislation. Any unwanted medicines should be returned to the pharmacy department for disposal.

Disposal of controlled drugs

It is important to ensure that any unwanted or expired stocks of CDs are disposed of in a safe manner to minimise the risk of them being inappropriately used or posing a public safety or environmental risk. The destruction of CDs is guided by the Misuse of Drugs Act 1971 and Misuse of Drugs Regulations 2001 (HMSO, 1971, 1973/2001). CDs can only be destroyed in the presence of a person authorised under these regulations to witness destruction. In a hospital setting, the authorised person is usually the pharmacist. When a CD is destroyed, it needs to be entered in the CD record book and witnessed by another healthcare professional, such as a registered nurse. CDs are placed in waste containers once they are **denatured**. This process renders the medicine irretrievable. **Denaturing kits** are available for this purpose.

Activity 5.7 *Evidence-based practice and research*

Consider the predominant group of patients you will be caring for during your nursing course. Identify at least two medicines that are stored:

(a) at room temperature;
(b) in a fridge;
(c) in a CD cupboard.

An outline answer is provided at the end of the chapter.

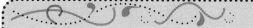

Chapter summary

This chapter has explored issues associated with the safe administration of medicines. It discusses the vital checks that must be made before your patients receive their medicines. The importance of accurate documentation is also highlighted as it is recognised that poor, inaccurate or incomplete documentation can result in medicine errors. Anaphylaxis, a medical emergency, is discussed with consideration as to why it occurs, how it manifests in your patient and how it is treated. We have explored the importance of reporting errors that occur in medicines management and how such reporting can be of benefit to current and future patients. Specific measures relevant to infection control precautions in the preparation, dispensing and administration stages of medicines management have been identified. The problems associated with polypharmacy are also discussed, as are measures to reduce its consequences to your patients. The concept of self-administration of medicines has also been explored with a particular focus on the importance of accurate patient assessment. Finally, the role of the nurse and the pharmacist in the ordering, receiving, storing and disposing of medicines has been discussed and issues relevant to controlled drugs have also been highlighted. Throughout this chapter there has been a focus on the roles and responsibilities of the registered nurse and other registered healthcare practitioners. You must remember that, as a student nurse, while you are not accountable professionally, you are accountable legally at all times for your actions or omissions, just like every other member of the general public.

Activities: brief outline answers

Activity 5.1 Types of errors and reasons for them (page 115)

Errors	Why?
Wrong medicine administered.	Prescription illegible. Similar packaging to another medicine. Similar medicine name to another medicine.
Wrong patient administered medicine.	Incorrect identification/non-identification of the patient.
Wrong dose of medicine given to patient.	Wrong dose prescribed. Prescription illegible. Incorrect dose calculated and dispensed.
Wrong route for administration of medicine.	Wrong route prescribed. Prescription illegible. Incorrect route read.
Wrong time for medicine to be administered.	Wrong time prescribed. Prescription illegible. Incorrect time read.
Wrong preparation for medicine to be administered, e.g. mixed in a wrong solution.	Wrong preparation dispensed from pharmacy. Nurse prepared medicine incorrectly.

Patient receives medicine they are allergic to.	No allergy recorded on prescription chart. Medicine incorrectly prescribed. No allergy recorded on patients wristband. Patient not asked if they had allergies. Nurse unaware that administered medicine contained a substance the patient was allergic to.
Nurse unaware that the medicine may cause ill effects due to the patient's current/ underlying health condition.	Medicine inappropriately prescribed. Poor knowledge regarding the patient's condition and/ or the medicine being administered.
Patient unaware of what medicine they are taking, therefore informed consent not adequately obtained.	Nurse does not ask permission and explain to the patient that they are being administered their medicines. Nurse does not ascertain the patient's understanding of their medical condition and the medicines they are taking in relation to it.

Activity 5.2 Confirming patients' identity (page 117)

(a) Patient is unable to understand or speak English.
(b) Babies or very young children will not have developed particular comprehension or verbal communication skills.
(c) Unconscious patients will be unable to respond verbally.
(d) Patients who have had strokes may have their speech affected, so may be unable to respond coherently or accurately.
(e) Patients with speech difficulties may not be able to articulate their details clearly.
(f) Patients may have cognitive impairment, for example head injuries, dementia or may be drowsy after a general anaesthetic.

Activity 5.3 Failure to sign for medicines (page 119)

(a) If the dose is inadvertently repeated, Alice will receive too much of the intended dose of the medicine. She may experience unpleasant or serious side effects as a result. Being so young she will not be able to articulate how she is feeling, so it may be difficult to ascertain fully what the side effects are.
(b) If the dose is not given and it was not given beforehand, Alice will not receive the dose of the medicine she should have had. This may have consequences for her medical condition.

Activity 5.4 Description of incident (page 125)

(a) This was an actual harm incident because Mrs Sullivan was given the wrong dose of medicine. While she does not appear to have suffered any ill effects from it, it was still an unplanned event that was not prevented.
(b) Three examples of what you could have written are:
  – The patient was administered the wrong dose of the medicine by Staff Nurse Decoats.
  – Mrs Sullivan was given too much of the prescribed medicine.
  – During the 8 a.m. medicine round Mrs Bridget Sullivan inadvertently received an incorrect dose of dihydrocodeine.

Activity 5.5 Refusal to take medicines (pages 130–1)

(a) Reasons why Jacob refuses his lunchtime medicines could include:
  – he may be hypoglycaemic and confused;
  – he may be distracted by activity in the day room;

- he may have difficulty in multi-tasking, e.g. being expected to take medicines, perhaps have lunch, while TV is on in the background and other patients are talking;
- he may be embarrassed about taking medicines in front of other patients;
- he may be experiencing unpleasant side effects associated with his medicines; he may not know what the medicines are for.

(b) What you could do to ensure Jacob takes his medicines includes:
- asking the interprofessional team to review his medicines regime;
- monitoring his blood glucose level just in case he is hypo/hyperglycaemic;
- taking blood samples for renal clearance; he may have toxic levels of one of the medicines in his circulatory system or he may be dehydrated – both of these conditions may cause him to be confused and agitated;
- ascertaining his knowledge re his medicines;
- asking if he is experiencing any side effects;
- administering his medicines by his bedside where he is less distracted by his surroundings.

Activity 5.6 Patient assessment and levels (page 134)

(a) It is likely that Priya would be assessed as level 3. This is because she is capable of accepting full responsibility for keeping her medicines safely stored. She is likely to remember when she should take her medicines.

(b) Priya is likely to be assessed as level 1 or 2. This will depend on how drowsy and stable she is after her general anaesthetic and operation. Patients who are under the influence of general anaesthesia or who are acutely ill will not be able to accept total responsibility for the storage and administration of their medicines.

(c) Moira will be assessed as level 3. She is capable of accepting full responsibility for keeping her daughter's medicines safely stored. She is likely to remember when her daughter needs to take her medicines.

(d) Harrison is likely to be assessed as level 1 or 2. This is due to his poor sight and short-term memory.

(e) Derek is likely to be assessed as level 1 or 2. He may be perfectly capable of storing his medicines safely and know what time they should be taken. However, as he has a history of alcohol and drug misuse he cannot be given total custody of his medicines.

Activity 5.7 Storage of medicines (page 136)

Examples include:

(a) thyroxine, amlodopine;
(b) insulin, amoxicillin suspension;
(c) morphine, fentanyl.

It is useful to refer to the instruction sheet that is supplied with medicines. This details the conditions in which the medicines should be stored.

Knowledge review

Now that you've worked through the chapter, how would you rate your knowledge of the following topics?

	Good	Adequate	Poor
1. Role of the nurse in the administration of medicines.			
2. Managing anaphylaxis.			
3. Adverse incident reporting.			
4. Infection control precautions in medicines management.			
5. Polypharmacy.			
6. Self-administration of medicines.			
7. Ordering, receiving, storing and disposing of medicines.			

Where you're not confident in your knowledge of a topic, what will you do next?

Further reading

Dimond, B (2004) Medicinal products and self-administration of medicines. *British Journal of Nursing*, 13(2): 101–3.

This is an interesting article detailing the legal aspects of self-administration of medicines.

Dougherty, L and Lister, S (eds) (2007) Drug administration: general principles, in *The Royal Marsden Hospital Manual of Clinical Nursing Procedures: Student edition*, 7th edition. Oxford: Wiley-Blackwell.

This chapter provides a useful insight into many aspects of medicines management.

Planton, J and Edlund, BJ (2010) Strategies for reducing polypharmacy in older adults. *Journal of Gerentological Nursing*, 36(1): 8–12.

This article details the implications of polypharmacy for the older patient and what can be done to minimise its impact.

Useful websites

www.mhra.gov.uk

Access to this website enables you to view the role and work of the Medicines and Healthcare products Regulatory Agency. You can report an adverse reaction to a medicine through the Yellow Card reporting system through this website.

www.npc.co.uk/mm

This website allows you access to the National Prescribing Centre. It takes you to their medicines management site, where you can view a variety of case scenarios related to medicines management issues. Open the five-minute guides for an overview of relevant issues and try the quizzes to test your knowledge.

Chapter 6
Medicines management in field-specific care environments

continued . . . •••

care environment and its location, can affect health, illness, health outcomes and public health priorities and take this into account in planning and delivering care.

6. All nurses must practise safely by being aware of the correct use, limitations and hazards of common interventions, including nursing activities, treatments, and the use of medical devices and equipment. The nurse must be able to evaluate their use, report any concerns promptly through appropriate channels and modify care where necessary to maintain safety. They must contribute to the collection of local and national data and formulation of policy on risks, hazards and adverse outcomes.

Domain 4: Leadership, management and team working

7. All nurses must work effectively across professional and agency boundaries, actively involving and respecting others' contributions to integrated person-centred care. They must know when and how to communicate with and refer to other professionals and agencies in order to respect the choices of service users and others, promoting shared decision making, to deliver positive outcomes and to coordinate smooth, effective transition within and between services and agencies

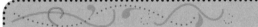

NMC Essential Skills Clusters

This chapter will address the following ESCs:

Cluster: Medicines management

All areas within this cluster are touched on in this chapter, to demonstrate how they might apply within each field of practice.

Chapter aims

By the end of this chapter, you should be able to:

- discuss relevant policies, legislation and evidence-based practice in relation to medicines management in specific care environments;
- explore the principles of medicines management in field-specific environments;
- understand the purpose of medical devices in an adult care environment;
- provide an overview of some common medical conditions;
- describe the medicines management care aspects for patients with specific medical conditions.

Introduction

As we have seen from previous chapters, it is important to get medicines management right for our patients. Their correct administration is a key element of care in all fields of nursing. The safe and effective use of medicines in all patient groups can be achieved through an evidence-based interprofessional approach involving nurses, nursing students, doctors, pharmacists and other healthcare professionals. Chapter 7 will explore the specific roles of key healthcare professionals in medicines management. This chapter will explore issues relating to medicines management in field-specific environments. It is not intended that this chapter will cover every aspect of medicines management relevant to each field of nursing; indeed, many issues have been covered in preceding chapters. Just a selection of issues has been chosen for each patient group. Even if you have already chosen your field of practice, we would encourage you to read the whole chapter, as it is important to understand medicines management issues in other fields. This is not only to enable you to understand the responsibilities of your colleagues and therefore how to work with them interprofessionally, but also so that you understand how to deliver core care to your patients regardless of their age or condition, as is made clear from the NMC *Standards* (2010a) outlined at the start of this chapter. This chapter is intended to be used by you early in your course so that you can start to understand the field-specific issues that you will come across. Further books in the series address medicines management for each field in more detail.

First, we shall explore the management of adult patients who receive their medicines via medical devices. Diabetes is a medical condition on the increase, partly due to unhealthy lifestyles. We shall discuss how adult patients can have their conditions best managed by pharmacological means. Patients with mental health issues require careful consideration and care tailored to meet their individual needs. Pain management will be considered as it can at times be difficult to treat effectively for such patients, particularly those who are taking illegal substances for recreational purposes. The medical condition that we shall explore for patients with mental health problems is schizophrenia. We shall discuss how this condition is controlled through pharmacological interventions.

Next, we shall explore further the issue of gaining informed consent in the patient with learning disabilities and how epilepsy can be managed in these patients. Ensuring children are given the correct dose of medicines is very important and we shall focus on why this is necessary and the consequences of not getting the dose right. It can at times be difficult to administer medicines to children and we shall explore some measures to take to ensure that children receive their medicines as intended. Asthma will be the medical condition discussed and its pharmacological management.

Adult nursing

Adult nursing is by far the largest field of practice of nursing. This is because of the vast age range of patients you will care for. Within such a varied age group you will encounter many patients with a diversity of illnesses and healthcare needs. These will be met in many different clinical settings, by a vast range of healthcare specialists. The different fields of nursing will at times need to work together to ensure that patients with complex healthcare needs are cared for by suitably experienced professionals. The many different medicines you will come across, coupled with the knowledge you need to acquire to administer them safely to your patients, may appear quite daunting. In this section we will consider some of the issues relevant to medicines management that you will come across while looking after adult patients. We will focus on how to care for a patient who is receiving medicines via medical devices and the pharmacological management of a patient with diabetes.

Managing medical devices

Medical devices encompass any equipment that is used in the delivery of healthcare. For example, electronic **sphygmomanometers**, used to measure your patients' blood pressure, **cardiac monitors**, used to monitor your patients' heart rate and rhythm, and even electric beds are just some of the different types of medical devices you will frequently see in the clinical setting.

You will encounter medical devices in all fields of nursing; adult nursing is just one field where you will see them used on a regular basis. When dealing with medicines we come across different types of medical devices. The most commonly used are **infusion devices**, which are designed to deliver a specific amount of fluid or medicine over a set period of time via different routes. These routes include intravenous, subcutaneous, epidural and nasogastric; you may wish to go back to Chapter 3 (see pp78–9) to recap on what these routes entail. Medicines can be infused using a syringe or a bag of fluids. There is a variety of devices available to assist in the delivery of medicines to your patients.

Gravity infusion devices

These devices are entirely dependent on gravity to deliver the infusion therapy. Put simply, they consist of an administration set containing a roller clamp and a drip chamber, which assists in regulating the flow rate of the infusion. The accuracy of the flow is dependent on the ability of the nurse to set it at the correct rate, using a simple mathematical formula (see Chapter 1, pp37–8). It can also be affected by factors such as changes in venous pressure, the position of your patient and the height of the infusion bag. Because of the risk of the unreliability of these devices, they should only be used for medicines or fluids where the risk of adverse effects is negligible or where your patient's medical condition does not give cause for concern (Dougherty and Lister, 2008).

Drip rate pumps

These pumps are simple battery- or mains-operated devices. They work by counting the number of drops per minute using a 'magic eye' or electronic drop counter. They do not have a pumping mechanism and therefore do not control the rate the infusion is running at. At best they provide a good estimate that the infusion is running to time. They are now no longer used in practice due to the errors that can occur (Lee, 2010).

Volumetric pumps

These electronic or battery-operated pumps require the rate of the infusion to be set in millilitres per hour. Unlike drip rate pumps, they do have a pumping action and are therefore able to overcome changes in venous pressure and offer accuracy in the delivery rate of an infusion (Dougherty and Lister, 2008).

Syringe pumps

You will come across a variety of syringe pumps in the clinical area. These devices enable relatively low volumes of medicines to be delivered at low infusion rates. This is important when administering medicines that have a narrow therapeutic range, such as insulin or heparin. Syringe drivers are often used in **palliative care** to deliver, typically, analgesics and/or anti-emetics to patients. You may come across older versions of these pumps that are set to deliver medicine volumes by distance (measured in millimetres per hour). Newer versions are set to deliver medicines in millilitres per hour.

Other types of syringe pumps include **patient-controlled analgesia (PCA) pumps**. These devices can be programmed to deliver a set amount of medicine over a certain period of time. They also allow for a maximum dose to be infused within a set period. They offer individual control to the patient, whereby the patient can operate the pump to deliver analgesia as and when they require it (this is known as a **bolus dose**). One of the most commonly used medicines in PCAs is morphine.

Activity 6.1   *Reflection*

List the types of medicines you have seen being delivered via a medical device. What type of device is used for each of the medicines you have listed? You may wish to list your answers under the following headings: 'Medicine' and 'Type of device'.

An outline answer is provided at the end of the chapter.

As a nursing student you will not be permitted to administer medicines via a medical device, as this usually involves additional training once you register as a qualified nurse. However, you should make available every opportunity to observe the setting up of these devices. That way you should acquire the confidence and competence to report to a registered nurse if you suspect a medical device has been incorrectly set up or if it malfunctions.

The Medicines and Healthcare products Regulatory Agency (MHRA), an executive agency of the Department of Health, is responsible for checking that all medicines and medical devices are safe to use. It is important to note that no medicine or device is totally risk-free, but the MHRA works to ensure that appropriate standards of quality, performance, effectiveness and safety are met (MHRA, 2010). All medicine errors that occur using medical devices should be reported to the MHRA. Over-infusion of medicines and fluids, which is reported frequently, often leads to patient harm or even death. Between 1990 and 2000 there were 1,495 errors reported involving medical devices in the UK (Medical Devices Agency, 2003). The majority of errors were classed as 'user error'. Causes of user error include:

- administration set or syringe not loaded correctly;
- wrong rate of infusion set;
- not confirming the set rate;
- not confirming the syringe size;
- confusing the pump type;
- not stopping the infusion correctly;
- configuration of the pump.

Diabetes

Diabetes is a **metabolic condition** characterised by an imbalance between how the body either produces or utilises **insulin**. There are several different types of this condition, with the main ones being **type 1** and **type 2 diabetes**. You may be familiar with other terms used to denote these types. Type 1 is also known as **insulin-dependent diabetes mellitus** and type 2 is also known as **non-insulin-dependent diabetes mellitus**. Following the intake of food, carbohydrates are broken down into glucose. Glucose is then absorbed into the bloodstream, and the resultant increase in blood glucose levels stimulate secretion of insulin by the pancreas. Insulin is a hormone produced in the **beta cells** of the **islets of Langerhans** in the pancreas. It is needed by most cells to enable glucose to enter them for energy. The cells are able to use the glucose, which then lowers glucose levels in the blood. When the body detects lowered blood glucose levels it decreases the secretion of insulin. If insulin production is lowered or absent, glucose will not be able to enter the cells. This will result in high levels of glucose in the bloodstream, which is known as **hyperglycaemia**. If insulin is secreted in large amounts this will allow more glucose to enter the cells and leave low levels of glucose in the bloodstream, which is known as **hypoglycaemia**. Excess glucose that the cells do not require is stored in the liver as glycogen. When the cells require energy, glycogen is converted into glucose. Fat and proteins can also be converted into glucose. This is a very simplified account of how the body is able to use glucose for energy. To learn more about this process you should refer to an anatomy and physiology textbook.

Differences between type 1 and type 2 diabetes

It is estimated that 5–15 per cent of all diabetes cases are type 1, and type 2 accounts for 85–95 per cent of all cases (Diabetes UK, 2010a, b). Type 2 diabetes is on the increase due to unhealthy lifestyles. Being overweight, lack of exercise and unhealthy diets are just some of the factors that put an individual at increased risk of developing the condition. An increase in type 2 diabetes in children is also associated with these risk factors. Table 6.1 outlines the key differences between type 1 and type 2 diabetes.

People with diabetes will experience some of the following signs and symptoms:

- passing increased amounts of urine (**polyuria**), especially at night time;
- increased thirst (**polydipsia**);

Type 1	Type 2
Signs and symptoms obvious and develop quite quickly, usually over a few weeks.	Signs and symptoms not so obvious.
No insulin produced.	Some insulin produced or insulin not able to be used by the body.
Usually appears in childhood or before 40 years of age.	Incidence increases with age, usually over 40 years of age.
Treated by insulin.	Tablets and/or insulin required to treat condition.

Table 6.1: Key differences between type 1 and type 2 diabetes

- increased fatigue and lethargy;
- unintentional weight loss;
- increased episodes of thrush;
- cuts and wounds slow to heal;
- blurred vision.

Pharmacological management of diabetes

There are essentially two different pharmacological treatments available for diabetes. The type of diabetes and the effect the condition has had on insulin production or its utilisation in the body will determine what treatment is used. Regardless of treatment choice, you should always encourage your patients to adopt a healthy lifestyle, including a balanced diet and exercise, both of which are important influences on how the condition is managed. Type 1 diabetes is treated with insulin and type 2 diabetes is sometimes treated with insulin, but often oral hypoglycaemic medicines are used.

Insulin

Insulin was originally extracted from the pancreas of cows (bovine) and pigs (porcine). These days insulin from animals is rarely used. Human insulin can be produced by modifying porcine insulin or by making human insulin using bacteria. It works by enabling glucose to enter the body cells, thereby lowering blood glucose levels. It also suppresses liver glucose production. For patients with both types of diabetes mellitus, insulin therapy enables them to control their blood glucose levels. It helps to reduce the onset of hyperglycaemia and also reduces the development of conditions such as cardiovascular disease, visual problems (for example **diabetic retinopathy**), poor wound healing, infection, renal impairment and poor peripheral circulation, which can, for example, lead to decreased sensation in the hands and feet. Insulin cannot be administered by the oral route because it would be destroyed by the stomach. It therefore needs to be administered via the intravenous or subcutaneous route.

Types of insulin

Short-acting

Short-acting insulin (also known as rapid-acting) has a relatively quick onset of action. There are different types of short-acting insulin. These include soluble insulin and rapid-acting human insulin analogues.

Soluble insulin (also called neutral insulin) has a clear appearance and is usually injected 15–30 minutes before mealtimes to control the rise in blood glucose levels that occur after food is eaten. When injected subcutaneously, it works within 30–60 minutes. It reaches its peak concentration in the bloodstream in two to four hours and its effects can last for up to eight hours. It is used in diabetic emergencies such as **diabetic ketoacidosis** and when a patient is having surgery.

Rapid-acting human insulin analogues have a cloudy appearance and a more rapid onset of action and shorter duration than soluble insulin. Types of this insulin include insulin aspart, insulin glulisine and insulin lispro. They are also useful for diabetic emergencies and at times of surgery. They have a lower associated risk of hypoglycaemia than soluble insulin.

If your patient has either type 1 or type 2 diabetes (controlled with oral medicines), they will require a continuous infusion of short-acting insulin prior to and during a surgical procedure. This will be administered via an infusion device, such as one discussed earlier in the chapter, via the intravenous route. It is important that you monitor your patient's blood glucose levels regularly, and the rate of insulin being administered will need to be adjusted according to their blood glucose level reading. Remember that, while you may be able to take your patient's blood glucose levels (subject to your individual hospital Trust protocol and university guidelines), you will not be allowed to alter the rate that the insulin is running at; this must always be done by a registered nurse.

Intermediate and long-acting

These insulins work in about one to two hours after subcutaneous administration. They reach their maximum effect at between four and twelve hours. Their duration of action lasts between 16 and 35 hours. Some of these insulins are given once a day, while others are given twice daily. These types of insulin include isophane insulin, insulin zinc suspension, protamine zinc insulin, insulin glargine and insulin determir. They are useful for patients who experience fluctuations in their blood glucose levels, particularly early in the morning. These insulins can also be mixed with short- or rapid-acting insulins. This helps to reduce the number of times a patient has to self-inject if they require both types. It also enables a continuous supply of insulin to be present in the blood to control entry of glucose into the cells.

Side effects of insulin

Both hypoglycaemia and hyperglycaemia can occur if there is a mismatch between the blood glucose level and the amount of insulin administered, or if the patient misses a dose or a meal or undertakes strenuous exercise. A condition called **lipodystrophy** can also occur. This effect is localised to the injection site. Subcutaneous fat in the injection site is dissolved by the insulin, causing the skin in that area to be depressed or indented (**lipoatrophy**) or it can cause a swelling of subcutaneous fat deposits (**lipohypertrophy**). It is for this reason that you should always encourage your patient to regularly change the site where they inject themselves with insulin. The patient can also become resistant to insulin, due to antibodies resistant to insulin forming in the blood. This causes the injected insulin to be destroyed in the blood. The patient requires a higher dose of insulin to bring about the desired effect.

Delivery devices

Insulin can be delivered by conventional methods, that is, needle and syringe, or by injection pens that hold the insulin in a cartridge so that a metered dose is delivered. Some patients require a continuous infusion of insulin, particularly in times of critical illness or during a surgical procedure, and so will use one of the infusion devices as outlined earlier in the chapter.

As a student nurse you will be involved under the direct supervision of a registered nurse in administering subcutaneous insulin to your patients. This may involve you preparing the insulin and equipment necessary to administer the insulin or it may require you to supervise your patient in their self-administration of the medicine.

Activity 6.2   *Communication*

Try the following exercise to test your understanding of the use of insulin in a patient with type 1 diabetes.

Semaj Bhati is a 19-year-old student with type 1 diabetes. He is attending at the outpatients' clinic for a routine check-up with the diabetic nurse specialist. After a discussion with Semaj the following issues have come to light.

- Semaj admits to binge drinking usually on two nights a week.
- He plays basketball for his university's team and trains two evenings a week, with a match usually on a Saturday morning. He also enjoys weight training at the gym.
- He admits to regularly missing meals due to his busy lifestyle.
- He tells you he usually injects insulin into his arm.

What advice would you give Semaj about his current lifestyle and how to administer his insulin?

You may need to refer to a physiology textbook and also a clinical skills book to help you answer this question.

An outline answer of what you might have considered is at the end of the chapter.

Oral antidiabetic medicines

Oral antidiabetic medicines are used to treat type 2 diabetes in conjunction with following a healthy lifestyle, which involves restricting energy and carbohydrate intake and increasing physical exercise. The most common medicines are sulphonylureas and biguanides. Some others include thiazolidinediones, meglitinides and acarbose.These medicines are administered either as a once-daily dose or in divided doses. They should be taken with or immediately after meals.

Sulphonylureas

These medicines are used when the pancreas is still able to produce some insulin. They work by stimulating the release of insulin from the pancreas. They do this by binding to potassium channels on beta cells to increase the secretion of insulin. To recap on the principles of pharmacology, go back to Chapter 3. These medicines also inhibit fat and proteins being converted to glucose in the liver and increase insulin receptors on cells to enable the cells to take in more insulin. Examples of these medicines include chlopropamide, glibenclamide, glicazide, glimepiride, glipizide and tolbutamide. As with all medicines, there is a possibility that your patient may experience some adverse effects. These are outlined in Table 6.2.

Biguanides

Biguanides work by decreasing the production of glucose and increasing the amount of glucose that enters cells. They also decrease the production of glucose in the liver. They require enough insulin to be present in the blood as they do not stimulate insulin release from the pancreas. Metformin is the only type of biguanide. It is recommended for patients with type 2 diabetes who are overweight and is the most commonly used antidiabetic medicine (Galbraith et al., 2007). Some adverse effects of the medicine are detailed in Table 6.2.

Thiazolidinediones

The mode of action of these medicines reduces insulin resistance, which is a common problem in type 2 diabetes. Pioglitazone and rosiglitazone are medicines in this class. There are several contraindications to their use. For example, they should not be used on patients who have heart conditions. More potential adverse effects are listed in Table 6.2.

Other antidiabetics

Other medicines used to treat diabetes include acarbose, which works by delaying the absorption of carbohydrates; and neteglinide and repaglinide, which stimulate the release of insulin. Some antidiabetic medicines are used in combination with insulin or other antidiabetic medicines. You should refer to a BNF or a pharmacology textbook to read more about these medicines and others used but not listed above.

Medicine	Some common adverse effects
Sulphonylureas	Hypoglycaemia, weight gain, nausea, vomiting, diarrhoea, skin reactions, bone marrow depression, **hyponatraemia, jaundice, hepatitis**
Biguanides	**Lactic acidosis**, nausea and vomiting
Thiazolidinediones	Oedema, anaemia, weight gain, exacerbated heart conditions

Table 6.2: Some common adverse effects of oral antidiabetic medicines

Mental health nursing

You will come across people of all ages who experience mental health issues. While most patients will easily be able to manage their conditions with the aid of medicines, you will care for those who will give you more complex issues to consider. This section will focus on areas of medicine management that can pose some tricky situations for you. We shall look at pain management in patients with a history of drug misuse and how, at times, their pain may not be adequately managed due to misconceptions among healthcare professionals.

Pain management in the drug misuse patient

An area of concern in medicines management for those with mental health issues is the correct management of their pain. Some patients may have difficulty in clearly expressing the pain they are experiencing. All patients should have their pain assessed, taking into account the use of pain assessment tools, recognition of physiological signs, and verbal and non-verbal expressions of pain.

Activity 6.3   *Reflection*

List the various signs you may see in a patient who is experiencing uncontrolled pain. You may wish to provide your list in a table with four headings: 'Physiological signs', 'Physical signs', 'Verbal signs' and 'Non-verbal signs'.

An outline answer is provided at the end of the chapter.

Individuals who have misused or are misusing opioids are at increased risk of having their pain control mismanaged. Nurses worry that patients will become addicted to the opioids and are using them to feed this perceived addiction rather than to control their pain. This is a misconception held by some healthcare professionals. In actual fact, people who have misused opioids often find that they need higher doses to control their pain. This is because their bodies are used to certain levels of opioids and, in order to actually experience the pain-relieving properties of the medicine, they need much more in their systems. You should refer to a physiology textbook to familiarise yourself with pain theories. The fear and frustration of not having their pain adequately controlled can often lead to patients becoming angry and venting their frustrations on the nursing staff and other members of the interprofessional team.

Drug misusers also have a tendency to have other mental health problems; often it is these problems that have led them to misuse drugs in the first place. You must always ensure that patients you look after who have a history of drug misuse are afforded the same care and respect as all your other patients.

Drug misuse

The term **drug misuse** refers to the use of a substance that is not for the purpose consistent with legal or medical guidelines (WHO, 2010). It is estimated that approximately three million people in the UK take illicit drugs (Hoare and Flatley, 2008).

Drug addiction/dependence

The terms **drug addiction** and **drug dependence** are often used interchangeably and can be described as the result of repeated administration of a controlled drug (CD). The person becomes so dependent on that medicine that he or she has an overwhelming need to continue taking it (Galbraith et al., 2007). There are many different reasons why people use medicines other than for treating a medical condition. For example, such misuse has been reported in sport, where sportsmen and women want to enhance their performances or lose or gain body weight to enable them to qualify for competitions. These medicines usually include **anabolic agents** to increase muscle and muscle strength, reduce body fat and promote aggression. Diuretics are also used to dilute the concentration of a medicine in urine, so that any performance-enhancing substances are less likely to be detected during routine **dope testing**. Other medicines that are misused in sport include **narcotics**, **hormones** and **stimulants**.

The most commonly used medicines that are prone to misuse by the general public are usually opioids. Euphoria is one of the many effects of opioids and is the effect often sought by those who misuse them. If a doctor caring for a patient considers him or her to be addicted to either cocaine, pethidine, morphine, methadone or opium, the doctor must inform the Chief Medical Officer at the Home Office, giving details about the patient. Drug misuse has been found to be particularly prevalent in mental health settings (NICE, 2008).

Drug tolerance

Over time, tolerance to a drug can occur in which the body becomes resistant to the effects of a medicine. Increased doses are required to bring about a desired or therapeutic effect. People can develop a tolerance to opioids – the longer that opioids such as morphine are taken the more tolerant the body becomes to them. Such patients therefore require increased doses to enable their pain to be controlled. The doses these patients require are in some cases high enough to kill those who are not tolerant of the medicine. The management of pain in people who misuse medicines will often require an interprofessional approach, such as specialised input from the pain team. This is because tolerance of a medicine in such patients will require them to take higher doses of the medicine to control their pain. This is not without its dangers, however, as one of the main adverse effects of opioids is over-sedation and respiratory depression. The risk of developing these adverse effects will increase with larger doses.

Schizophrenia

Schizophrenia is a chronic mental health condition caused by an imbalance in mental function. It is linked to an abnormal function in **dopamine** pathways in the brain. Dopamine is a neurotransmitter found in the brain. It is involved in the coordination of motor and intellectual impulses and responses. Schizophrenia is usually characterised by **hallucinations** (seeing or hearing things that do not exist) or **delusions** (believing in things that are not true). Schizophrenia is a serious medical condition with about one in every 100 people experiencing at least one schizophrenic episode in their life. It usually starts in young adults. Because it derives from a Greek word that means 'split mind', it is a commonly held misconception that people with schizophrenia have split or dual personalities. Symptoms of the condition are divided into positive and negative conditions. Positive symptoms include hallucinations and delusions, while negative symptoms include lack of thoughts or function that you would expect to see in a healthy individual. Table 6.3 outlines the symptoms of the condition. Complete recovery from schizophrenia is unusual, but a considerable improvement in the patient's condition is achievable. The condition tends to manifest itself in times of stress and is thought to be made worse by the use of illicit drugs such as cannabis and ecstasy.

Pharmacological methods to treat schizophrenia

For many patients the symptoms of schizophrenia can be relieved by dopamine-blocking medicines. **Typical antipsychotic medicines** (or **neuroleptics**) are used as soon as a diagnosis has been made. It is vital that patients are able to comply with the medicine regime, otherwise relapses in their condition will occur. If your patient is unable to comply with taking their medicines, **depot injections** are a useful alternative. It usually takes about four to six weeks before the effectiveness of the medicine can be fully assessed. If the patient does not respond to these medicines, the use of **atypical antipsychotic drugs** (**AADs**) may be considered. Both

Positive symptoms	Negative symptoms
Hearing voices that do not exist.	Social withdrawal.
Seeing things that do not exist.	Lack of personal care.
Believing something or someone wants to hurt, mislead, manipulate or kill you.	Lack or flattening of emotions.
Believing you have imaginary power.	Poor motivation.
Delusions of grandeur.	Becoming increasingly uncommunicative.
Attaching undue or misguided significance to everyday occurrences.	Unable to enjoy things you used to.
Concentration problems.	
Acting in an unusual or bizarre manner.	
Thinking in a muddled or confused way.	

Table 6.3: Symptoms of schizophrenia (NHS, 2010b)

types of medicines work by interfering with the normal action of brain neurotransmitters, such as dopamine and their receptors. The response to these medicines will vary considerably between each patient and this is a reason why there are so many different medicines available to treat schizophrenia.

Typical antipsychotic medicines

Antipsychotic medicines include neuroleptics or typical antipsychotic medicines. Some people class these medicines as tranquillisers that are used to induce sleep or drowsiness. However, these medicines are used to calm down patients with schizophrenia and reduce the severe anxiety and agitation that such patients may experience. As a result, their aim is not to help patients go to sleep or make them drowsy. They appear to work best on the positive symptoms of schizophrenia (see Table 6.3). Medicines included in this class are phenothiazines, butyrophenones, diphenylbutylpiperidines, thioxanthenes and the substituted benzamides. Which one to choose very much depends on how much calming down the patient requires and the extent to which he or she may suffer from the adverse effects of the medicines. Common adverse effects are outlined in Table 6.5 on p156. The side effects are particularly associated with movement disorders in the body and face – **extrapyramidal** and **tardive dyskinesia** – which occur as a result of disturbances in nerve pathways from the brain stem to the spinal cord. This in turn has an effect on skeletal muscle.

Phenothiazines

These medicines have an antipsychotic effect and are helpful in reducing hallucinations, restlessness and agitation. They are divided into three main groups according to their sedative, extrapyramidal and **antimuscarinic effects** (see Table 6.4), with the medicines in group 3 having lesser sedative and antimuscarinic effects but more pronounced extrapyramidal effects.

Butyrophenones

These medicines include benperidol and haloperidol. Benperidol is particularly useful in controlling unacceptable antisocial sexual behaviour. Haloperidol is useful in treating patients who are in a very agitated state and are at risk of dangerous or violent behaviour.

Group 1	Group 2	Group 3
Chlorpromazine	Pericyazine	Fluphenazine
Levomepromazine	Pipotiazine	Perphenazine
Promazine		Prochlorperazine
		Trifluoperazine

Table 6.4: The phenothiazines

Diphenylbutylpiperidines

Pimozide is a medicine also used in the treatment of schizophrenia. **Electrocardiographs (ECGs)** should be taken prior to a patient commencing this medicine due to reports of unexplained deaths. Annual ECGs are recommended.

Thioxanthenes

Flupentixol and zuclopenthixol are useful for patients with schizophrenia. They can both be administered orally and via a depot injection, the latter being particularly useful for patients who are unable to comply with taking their medicines regularly.

Substituted benzamides

Sulpiride has fewer extrapyramidal effects than some other antipsychotic medicines. It also has a more specific dopamine-blocking action than some other medicines.

Atypical antipsychotic drugs (AADs)

These medicines should be used if typical antipsychotic medicines are ineffective and particularly in acute schizophrenic episodes when you are not able to discuss treatment with your patient. Table 6.5 lists the main adverse effects of these medicines. They produce fewer adverse effects, such as tremors, than typical antipsychotics, and work differently in that their mode of action is confined to the area of the brain concerned with schizophrenia. The atypical antipsychotics include amisulpride, aripiprazole, clozapine, olanzapine, quetiapine, risperidone and zotepine. They are more effective than typical antipsychotics in treating the negative symptoms of schizophrenia (see Table 6.3). A selection of these medicines is briefly discussed below.

Clozapine

Clozapine is useful for patients who are not responsive to or are unable to tolerate other antipsychotic medicines. Its use has been associated with an increased risk of **neutropenia** (a decrease in the number of white blood cells in the blood), so would limit a patient's ability to fight off an infection.

Risperidone

This medicine is useful for those who experience acute and chronic psychoses as part of their schizophrenia.

Aripiprazole

Aripiprazole works on both the positive and negative symptoms of schizophrenia.

Atypical psychotics are more costly than their typical psychotic counterparts and this is one reason why they are usually the second medicine of choice when treating schizophrenia.

Typical antipsychotics	Atypical antipsychotics
Parkinsonian symptoms, such as tremors.	Mild extrapyramidal effects.
Dystonia – abnormal face and body movements.	Weight gain.
Dyskinesia – abnormal body movements.	**Hyperlipidemia**.
Akathisia – restlessness, tension, panic, impatience and irritability.	Cardiac arrhythmias.
Tardive dyskinesia – involuntary rhythmic movements of jaw, tongue and face.	**Myocarditis**.
Hypotension.	Neutropenia (when clozapine is used).
Hypothermia and hyperthermia.	Hyperglycaemia.
	Type 2 diabetes.
	Sexual dysfunction.

Table 6.5: Common adverse effects of antipsychotic medicines

Activity 6.4   *Evidence-based practice and research*

Davindra Mahmood is a 27-year-old unemployed homeless man. He has been sleeping rough for the past three months. He has been diagnosed with schizophrenia. His mental health is deteriorating and he has not been taking his oral antipsychotic medicines as prescribed. His community mental health team have decided that he should be administered his medicine via a four-weekly depot injection.

Consider the advantages and disadvantages to Davindra of receiving his medicines in this way. You may wish to draw up a table with advantages in one column and disadvantages in the other.

An outline answer is provided at the end of the chapter.

More detailed information on the pharmacological actions of the medicines used to treat schizophrenia can be found in a good pharmacology textbook.

Learning disabilities nursing

Learning disabilities is an area of nursing that spans all the other fields of nursing. Approximately one million people in the UK have a learning disability (DH, 2001c). There is a great deal of research to support the notion that people with learning disabilities do not receive adequate healthcare and are not afforded the same opportunities to receive equal healthcare as the rest of the population. It is suggested that people with learning disabilities are 58 times more likely to die before the age of 50 years and four times more likely to die from a preventable cause of death compared to the general population (Hollins et al., 1998). You will encounter both adults and children with learning disabilities and mental health needs. Both physiological and psychological aspects of care need to be addressed in the patient with learning disabilities. Many people with learning disabilities used to live in institutions or long-stay hospitals, but these places have gradually closed down over the years, with the recognition that people with learning disabilities have a right to live in the community.

Obtaining informed consent for the patient with learning disabilities can be challenging, but not necessarily impossible. This section will address legal, ethical and professional issues associated with gaining consent and some practical measures will be discussed as to how to ensure the consent you gain from your patient for any treatment is valid. The management of epilepsy is an important consideration for those with learning disabilities, as is behavioural management. This section will explore the pharmacological methods used to treat and control the symptoms of epilepsy and behavioural issues.

Activity 6.5   *Evidence-based practice and research*

There are many reasons why people with learning disabilities experience inequalities in healthcare and shorter life expectancies. List the reasons why you think this occurs.

An outline answer is provided at the end of the chapter.

Informed consent

Informed consent has already been discussed broadly in Chapter 2. This section will focus on how it can be gained from the patient with learning disabilities. Practical measures that need to be considered in order to enhance your patients' understanding of any treatment they are being offered will also be explored.

Mental capacity/decision-making capacity

Under the Mental Capacity Act 2005, a person is deemed to have the mental capacity to agree to a treatment unless it can be proved otherwise (HMSO, 2005). It is wrong to make an assumption that a patient lacks the ability to give consent just because he or she has a learning disability. Consent is only deemed valid if it is given voluntarily by an appropriately informed individual who possesses the capacity to consent to a treatment or intervention (DH, 2007b). Mental capacity is key to an individual's level of autonomy in the care they receive. The Mental Capacity Act 2005 defines a lack of capacity as the inability to make a decision for oneself due to a temporary or permanent disturbance or impairment in the functioning of mind or brain. In order to ascertain whether your patients have the capacity to give informed consent, you must be satisfied that they are able to understand the information relevant to the decision they are being required to make; that they can retain that information; that they have the ability to use or weigh up the information as part of the decision-making process; and that they are able to communicate the decisions they make. This could be by speech or sign language, including activities such as blinking an eye or squeezing a hand.

Most patients with learning disabilities do have the ability to make decisions regarding their health and treatments. For some, though, it is how this information is conveyed to them that will influence their understanding and whether they agree to the proposed treatment.

Gaining valid informed consent

For any patient, and in particular the patient with learning disabilities, coming into hospital for treatment can be a daunting experience. This can be further exacerbated by the expectation from healthcare professionals that the patient must make decisions regarding his or her own care. In order to make the process informative and beneficial to the patient, information needs to be given in a way that your patient can understand. For example, you should use language and terms that your patient can understand, speaking clearly and at a steady pace. Some patients may also find it useful to look at pictures, diagrams or symbols to aid their understanding.

Consider the following true cases.

Case study

Emma, a 26-year-old lady with severe learning disabilities, died of cancer. Due to her communication difficulties and at times challenging behaviour, the hospital delayed treating her because they said she could not cooperate with treatment and could not give consent.

(Source: Mencap, 2007.)

Katherine was 30 years old when she was admitted to hospital with chest problems. She also suffered from severe epilepsy. Hospital staff forgot to administer her anti-epileptic medicine to her and she died after a prolonged fit.

(Source: Mencap, 2004.)

It must be remembered that any discrimination, intended or otherwise, against somebody because of their disability breaches the Disability Discrimination Act (DDA) 1995 (HMSO, 1995) and is therefore illegal.

Consenting on someone else's behalf

Legally, it is not permissible for somebody else to consent on behalf of a patient who lacks capacity. There are some exceptions, however, namely if they have lasting power of attorney or have been given the authority to make decisions as a court-appointed deputy. Generally, relatives, friends, doctors and other healthcare professionals cannot consent on behalf of a patient with learning disabilities who lacks capacity.

Activity 6.6   *Communication*

As a student nurse you are required to administer, under the direct supervision of a registered nurse, a medicine to Bill Watts that he has never taken before. Bill has learning disabilities. What measures should you take to ensure that you have obtained valid informed consent from him before you give him his medicine?

You may wish to obtain a copy of the Mental Capacity Act 2005 (HMSO, 2005) to assist you in answering this question.

An outline answer is provided at the end of the chapter.

It is important to remember that informed consent is not signified merely by a signature on a consent form or a compliant patient; it is a process that takes careful consideration and time to ensure that all parties are happy with the decision-making process.

Epilepsy

Epilepsy is a neurological condition that is characterised by recurrent seizures (Stokes et al., 2004). These seizures can range in length of duration and severity and are caused by electrical discharges in the brain. The discharge may be confined to one area of the brain causing **focal seizures**, characterised by an **aura**, or be more generalised, where the patient experiences brief seizures without convulsions (**petit-mal** or **absence seizures**). These seizures usually involve very brief periods of loss of consciousness, usually just a few seconds. Generalised seizures that begin in one area of the brain and quickly spread throughout both hemispheres can last for several minutes, causing **tonic-clonic convulsions** or **grand-mal seizures**. These seizures usually result in loss of consciousness, with the patient appearing tired and confused during the recovery period. The spread of the electrical discharge may be limited, resulting in **partial seizures**, which manifest as psychological disturbances such as mood swings or uncharacteristic behaviour. Where seizures become prolonged or recurrent, with the patient not recovering in between, the patient is said to be in **status epilepticus**. This condition is serious and requires emergency treatment.

While learning disabilities do not cause epilepsy or vice versa, it does appear to be more prevalent in those with learning disabilities compared to the rest of the population. Approximately 20–30 per cent of people with learning disabilities have epilepsy (Bernal, 2003), which is about 20 times higher than the general population (DH, 2008). Epilepsy can also be quite difficult to diagnose, since it can be mistaken for other behavioural issues that are seen in those with learning disabilities. For example, repetitive behaviour can be a sign of an epileptic seizure, but it is also a common trait in those with more severe forms of learning disability (Searson, 2008). Some people are born with epilepsy, while others go on to develop the condition in childhood, adolescence or adulthood.

There are three main categories of epilepsy. These are **symptomatic epilepsy**, where there is a known cause for the patient's epilepsy; **idiopathic epilepsy**, where a cause cannot be identified; and **cryptogenic epilepsy**, which is thought to be linked to brain damage and learning disabilities. The causes or factors linked to each are listed in Table 6.6.

Symptomatic	Idiopathic	Cryptogenic
Stroke Brain tumours **Cerebral palsy** Drug and alcohol misuse Birth defects Deprived of oxygen at birth **Meningitis** Head injuries	Genetic defects	Learning difficulties **Autism** Unusual **electroencephalogram (EEG)**

Table 6.6: Causes and factors of epilepsy (NHS, 2010a)

Medicines used in the treatment of epilepsy

There are many different types of medicines used to treat epilepsy. The treatment choice will depend on the type of seizure the patient experiences, their age, gender and any other medicines they are taking. Medicine dosage is kept as low as possible to minimise any unpleasant side effects, thereby promoting concordance by the patient with their medicines regime. The majority of medicines are administered once or twice daily. We shall take a brief look at some of the common medicines used to treat epilepsy. You should refer to the BNF to learn about other medicines for this condition not discussed in this chapter. The main adverse effects of the medicines discussed are listed in Table 6. 7.

Phenytoin

This medicine is particularly useful at treating patients who experience tonic-clonic seizures. It can also be used to treat partial seizures. It works by blocking sodium ions in nerve cell membranes. This reduces the excitability of nerve cells and prevents electrical discharge from spreading throughout the brain.

Carbamazepine

Carbamazepine is used in the treatment of tonic-clonic and partial seizures. Similarly to phenytoin, it works by blocking sodium ions in nerve cell membranes.

Sodium valproate

Sodium valproate is effective in managing all forms of epilepsy.

Ethosuximide

This medicine can be used to treat absence seizures.

Gabapentin and pregabalin

These are used in the management of partial seizures.

Phenobarbital

This medicine can be used for partial seizures and tonic-clonic seizures. It belongs to a group of medicines known as barbiturates, and it works by stabilising electrical impulses in the brain to prevent seizures.

Clonazepam

Clonazepam is sometimes used for tonic-clonic or partial seizures. It is also used for those patients who are in status epilepticus. It belongs to a class of medicines known as **benzodiazepines**.

Medicine	Some adverse effects
Phenytoin	Gum overgrowth **Hirsutism** Blurred vision
Carbamazepine	Cardiovascular disturbances Liver and kidney dysfunction Blurred vision Dizziness Nausea and vomiting
Sodium valproate	Liver toxicity Blood disorders Liver disorders **Pancreatitis**
Ethosuximide	Blood disorders
Gabapentin	Anxiety Diabetes mellitus Insomnia Nausea
Pregabalin	Severe congestive heart failure
Phenobarbital	Drowsiness Irritability
Clonazepam	Drowsiness Dizziness Blurred vision Tolerance (long term) Withdrawal symptoms **Alopecia**

Table 6.7: Adverse effects of anti-epileptic drugs (AEDs)

Epilepsy in a patient with learning disabilities is best managed by the use of a single anti-epileptic drug (AED). Sodium valproate and carbamazepine are the most commonly used AEDs in the treatment of epilepsy.

Activity 6.7   *Evidence-based practice and research*

(a) Using the BNF or another pharmacology textbook, list the common doses and the recommended frequency of administration for sodium valproate and carbamazepine.

(b) What are the benefits to the patient of taking these or similar medicines used to treat epilepsy?

An outline answer is provided at the end of the chapter.

Children's nursing

An important area of medicines management in children is ensuring that they receive the correct dose of medicine. While it is vital that you are competent at performing dosage calculations for all your patients, the consequences of underdosing and particularly those of overdosing will quickly become apparent in the child. Drug concordance is another area that at times can pose difficulties. It can be quite tricky trying to explain to a young child that an unpleasant-tasting medicine or a potentially painful injection will do them no harm. Asthma is a medical condition on the increase in children and we shall briefly explore what it is and the causes and then look at the pharmacological interventions used to treat asthma in children.

Getting the dose right

Unlike adults, where for many medicines one dose will be more or less the same for everybody, children respond differently to medicines. When calculating the right dose it is far more complex than simply, say, halving or quartering adult doses. We have seen from Chapter 1 that extra care needs to be taken when calculating children's medicines. Often doses are prescribed according to the child's body weight or body surface area. Considerations also need to be taken regarding the age and the stage of development of the child. You may wish to refer back to Chapter 3 to recap on the pharmacology of medicines. Table 6.8 outlines some of the differences between an adult and a child that should be taken into consideration when prescribing the correct dose of medicine.

As you can see, there are many physiological differences between adults and children and this is the reason why doses of medicine cannot be simply reduced proportionally by age.

Many medicines that are used to treat children are prescribed outside their product licence (see Chapter 2 on medicines legislation). This is because the majority of medicines in use only receive a licence for adult use once they have undergone rigorous testing and are deemed safe for use on humans. The majority of testing is carried out by clinical trials and it is not considered ethically

Differences	Caution
Lower levels of gastric acid.	Reduced ability of acid-based medicines to be absorbed in the stomach.
Thinner skin.	Topical medicines may be absorbed too quickly.
Poorer tissue perfusion.	Medicines less able to circulate to all areas of the body.
Less muscle mass.	May influence rate of absorption of medicine at injection site.
Lower levels of plasma protein.	Higher levels of unbound medicine in circulatory system.
Less adipose tissue.	Increased, but short-lasting, reaction to fat-soluble medicines.
Less enzymatic activity.	Medicines not broken down as quickly.
Slower glomerular filtration and blood flow to the kidneys (in children less than one year).	Slower clearance of medicines from the body.

Table 6.8: Key differences between adult and children relative to medicine dosages

viable to recruit children to such trials. Equally, it would not be ethical to withhold these medicines from children to treat their conditions. Therefore, most medicines used for children have not been tested on children. They rely very much on the skills, knowledge and expertise of the prescriber and those who administer their medicines to ensure that they receive the correct doses.

Activity 6.8   *Evidence-based practice and research*

Research a news story where a child received the wrong dose of medicine. Try to find out what, why and how the error happened. What were the consequences to the child? Using a BNF, find out the normal dose that the child in your news story should have received.

As this activity is designed to use your research skills, there is no outline answer provided at the end of this chapter.

Concordance

You will by now be familiar with the term 'concordance' and the factors that enable patients to either comply with their medicine regimen or disregard it. This section will pay particular attention to how children are enabled to take their medicines.

It is always better and easier to have a compliant child when administering medicines. As a paediatric nursing student you should involve children as much as possible in the medicine administration process. Building up a friendly and trusting relationship with the children will go a long way towards making them feel at ease with you. This in turn will make them more comfortable with taking their medicines. How much children are involved will depend on their age and level of understanding, family and guardian influences and other circumstances.

Administration stage

Oral route

It is far preferable, where possible, for children to be administered their medicines by the oral route. This usually causes less stress (and pain) for the child, is less time-consuming than other methods to prepare and administer, and is usually a less costly method (since less equipment is needed). This may simply involve placing a tablet directly on to the child's tongue or you may need to use a syringe, spoon, dropper or medicine cup. You must ensure that the child is sitting upright to avoid any possible risk of gagging, choking or aspirating when you administer the medicine. With very young children you should also ensure that their hands are placed away from the medicine container. You must never administer any medicines to children who are crying or sleeping, for risk of choking. Very young babies can be held in a semi-sitting position with their heads upright. Use a liquid preparation if possible because it is usually easier and quicker to dispense; but it will depend on the child's tolerance, his or her medical condition, the pharmacological action of the medicine and, in some cases, the volume of liquid that will need to be taken.

Children should not be rushed to take their medicines. You must allow them time, remaining fair but firm at all times. You should always witness that a child has taken and swallowed the medicine. For young babies, stroking the cheek or under the chin will encourage a sucking and swallowing reflex. Older children should be encouraged to take their medicines from a medicine pot or spoon rather than a syringe to reduce the medicalisation of medicines administration. It may also be useful (if permitted) to allow the child the opportunity to take a flavoured drink after the medicine has been administered to dilute or disguise any unpleasant taste.

Covert administration of medicines

In Chapter 2 we discussed covert administration of medicines; however, this has been predominantly based on the adult patient, with the NMC (2007a) offering clear guidance on if and when it should be considered.

In children's nursing it is a more common practice to crush tablets, open capsules and dissolve or hide them in food and drink than in adult nursing. It must be remembered that doing this makes the medicine unlicensed for use and the liability for any adverse consequences will devolve from the manufacturer to the prescriber and administrator of the medicine; in other words, you. It is accepted in children's nursing that there will be occasions when this happens. Care should be taken, including communication with the pharmacist and careful consideration of any manufacturer's instructions and advice. It is also advisable to ensure that any medicines crushed or dissolved are done so in small amounts of liquid or food. This is to ensure that the child takes the entire dose. If this practice is carried out, after careful consideration, you must be sure that the medicine's therapeutic properties are not changed as a result of the way it is administered.

Intramuscular and subcutaneous routes

Special consideration needs to be taken when administering medicines via injections to children. It is best practice when you are preparing any medicines for administration, particularly injections, to do it away from the child to minimise their distress. It is best to have two nurses involved in administering injections: one to keep the injection site still and distract the child. The preferred site for intramuscular injections is the **vastus lateralis** as the muscle is better developed here than at other sites. It is also important to be honest with children. There is little point in telling a child that an injection will not be painful when it is likely to cause some degree of discomfort; the child is less likely to agree to have it administered the next time. A better approach would be to explain, in language that is suitable to the child's age and developmental stage, that it will be uncomfortable but that the pain will not last for long. Factors that have been identified as causing pain when giving injections are:

- *the needle;*
- *the composition of the solution;*
- *the technique used;*
- *the speed at which the injection is administered;*
- *the amount of liquid administered.*

(Torrence, 1989)

To lessen the potential painful experience, psychological preparation such as giving the child the appropriate amount of information at the right level, and distraction therapy such as allowing the child to cuddle a favourite toy while the administration of the injection takes place should help. Ensuring that the child is in a comfortable position where the muscle to be injected is relaxed will also help. Freezing sprays or numbing creams, often referred to as 'magic creams' for younger children, applied to the skin site prior to the administration of the injection are also worth considering. Emla cream is a brand name topical medicine consisting of prilocaine and lidocaine (local anaesthetics) that can be applied under an occlusive dressing prior to administering an intramuscular injection, to numb the skin.

Self-administration of medicines

We have discussed self-administration of medicines in Chapter 5. The NMC also supports this activity in children; similarly to adult patients, this is dependent on their condition, age and level of understanding. For younger children it is recommended that parents/guardians play an active role in administering medicines to their children. This is important as children already have trusting relationships with these adults and may be more likely to listen to them and take their medicines. It also serves as a useful educational activity to ensure concordance with the medicine regime on discharge. Whichever method is used to administer medicine to a child, it must be remembered that the registered nurse will always remain accountable for any actions, omissions or consequences caused by the parent/guardian.

Asthma

Asthma is a chronic medical condition affecting about 1.1 million children in the UK (Asthma UK, 2010). It often starts in childhood, although people of any age can go on to develop the condition. It is thought to be an **autoimmune** condition where antibodies to common allergens are formed. When the patient is exposed to the allergen, inflammatory mediators such as histamine are released. Constriction of the bronchioles, spasm of the airways and swelling of the lining of the airways occur, resulting in the characteristic wheeze associated with asthma attacks. Other symptoms include coughing, shortness of breath and tightness in the chest. Such attacks can be triggered by things the patient is allergic to, such as pet hair or grass pollen. Other triggers include household dust, tobacco smoke, pollutants, the common cold, physical exertion, infections, cold air and emotional state. **Status asthmaticus** is a life-threatening condition where **bronchospasm** does not respond to treatment and air flow to the lungs is occluded. People with eczema appear to have an increased risk of developing asthma.

Pharmacological methods used to treat asthma

The pharmacological treatment of asthma consists of several different types of medicines. The main aim of medicines in asthma management is to prevent an asthma attack, or to relieve an attack. The classes of medicines commonly used are **bronchodilators**, **corticosteroids**, **cromoglicate**, **nedocromil** and **leukotriene receptor antagonists**. Oxygen may also be used in the management of asthma. However, this section will discuss pharmacological management only. There are various routes for administration, including inhalation, oral and parenteral.

Bronchodilators

Bronchodilators are used for the relief of asthma. A short-acting beta 2 agonist is used for the immediate relief of asthma. These medicines are inhaled and common ones are salbutamol or terbutaline. They are also useful immediately before exercise to prevent an attack induced by exercise. Long-acting beta 2 agonists are used for long-term asthma management and include formoterol and salemetarol. Common adverse effects are outlined in Table 6.9.

Inhalers are used to deliver a metered dose of the bronchodilator to the patient. In children the use of a **spacer** is recommended. This is because a spacer slows down the speed at which the medicine leaves the aerosol. The medicine is then stored in the spacer and the child has more time to inhale the medicine, compared to using the inhaler alone. Another advantage of using a spacer is that more medicine will enter the lungs, rather than hitting the back of the throat and being swallowed. Other devices available include a dry powder inhaler or a breath-actuated inhaler. Beta 2 agonists can also be administered via **nebulisers** or as an oral preparation. In life-threatening situations they can also be administered intravenously.

Corticosteroids

Corticosteroids work by reducing inflammation in the airway. This reduces oedema and the secretion of mucus into the airway. They help to prevent asthma attacks and should be used regularly. As with bronchodilators, they are usually administered via inhalation, although they can be taken orally and in emergency cases intravenously. Common corticosteroids used are beclometasone dipropionate, budenoside, fluticasone propionate and mometasone furoate. It is recommended that children under the age of 15 use a spacer device to inhale corticosteroids (NICE, 2000). Some common side effects are listed in Table 6.9.

Cromoglicate and nedocromil

Sodium cromoglicate and nedocromil sodium are used to prevent asthma attacks. When taken by inhalation they prevent the release of inflammatory mediators and so reduce the risk of an attack. Common adverse effects are listed in Table 6.9.

Leukotriene receptor antagonists

Leukotrienes are inflammatory molecules released by mast cells during an asthma attack and are responsible for the constriction of the bronchioles. Leukotriene receptor antagonists block the action of these inflammatory molecules and so reduce inflammation and bronchoconstriction. Montelukast and zafirlukast are medicines in this group that are used for the treatment of asthma. They are administered via the oral route. Common adverse reactions are listed in Table 6.9.

Now try the following activity to test your knowledge of the pharmacological management of asthma.

Medicine	Some adverse effects
Bronchodilators	Fine tremor; palpitations; headache; nervous tension; peripheral dilatation; tachycardia; arrhythmias; myocardial ischaemia; muscle cramps; angioedema; hypokalaemia.
Corticosteroids	Adrenal suppression; adrenal crisis and coma; possible growth restriction; hoarseness; candida of mouth and throat.
Cromoglicate and nedocromil	Unpleasant taste; coughing.
Leukotriene receptor antagonists	Headache; gastrointestinal disturbances; **hyperkinesia**; angioedema; skin reactions; hepatic disorder.

Table 6.9: Common adverse reactions of medicines used in asthma management

Activity 6.9   *Communication*

You are on placement at a GP surgery. The practice nurse is running an asthma management clinic for children. She has asked you to draw up a poster that would be suitable for children between the ages of 8 and 12 titled 'How to prevent an asthma attack'. What information would the practice nurse expect to see on your poster?

An outline answer is provided at the end of the chapter.

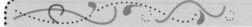

Chapter summary

This chapter had explored a variety of issues and the pharmacological management of some medical conditions specific to each of the four fields of nursing. From reading this chapter you will have gained an insight into the types of medical devices used to administer medicines to your patients and some of the potential problems that can arise from using this equipment. The use of insulin and hypoglycaemic medicines has also been discussed in the treatment of an adult patient with diabetes mellitus. Treating pain in a patient with a history of drug misuse and the misconceptions surrounding the use of opioids in managing pain have been highlighted. Schizophrenia has been briefly explored, as have the medicines used to manage its symptoms. The importance of ensuring that patients with learning disabilities are able to be active partners in their care and are afforded equal opportunities as other patients in receiving treatment that they are able to understand and give informed consent to have also been explored. You have learnt that people with learning disabilities have an increased risk of developing certain illnesses and medical conditions, and that epilepsy appears to be more prevalent in this group of people. Medicines used to treat epilepsy have been identified. Finally, the importance of ensuring that children receive the correct dosages of medicines and tips to improve concordance have been explored. Asthma, a common medical condition in children, and its management have also been identified.

Completion of the activities and undertaking additional reading into these important areas of medicines management will assist you in acquiring the necessary proficiency for entry into your field of nursing.

Activities: brief outline answers

Activity 6.1 Medical devices (page 145)

Medicine	Type of device
Heparin	Syringe pump
Insulin	Syringe pump
Morphine	Syringe pump (patient-controlled analgesia – PCA)
	Syringe driver
Dextrose saline	Gravity infusion device
Metoclopramide	Syringe driver
Normal saline with potassium chloride	Volumetric pump
Vancomycin	Volumetric pump

Activity 6.2 Use of insulin (page 149)

- Semaj should be discouraged from binge drinking as this can cause hypoglycaemia.
- He should be advised of the importance of taking regular meals to maintain satisfactory levels of carbohydrate and insulin to regulate blood glucose levels.
- He should not be injecting insulin into his arm as there is little if any subcutaneous tissue; there is a risk that Semaj will inject into a muscle. Semaj also lifts weights and an increase in physical or muscle activity will cause insulin to be absorbed much more quickly into the bloodstream.

Activity 6.3 Signs of pain (page 151)

Physiological signs	Physical signs	Verbal signs	Non-verbal signs
Increased blood pressure	Guarding of area where pain is located	Crying	Depression
Increased pulse rate	Pale skin	Shouting	Appearing withdrawn
Increased temperature	Goosebumps	Groaning	
Increased or decreased respirations	Dilated pupils	Cursing, swearing	
	Nausea and vomiting		

Activity 6.4 Depot injections for schizophrenia (page 156)

Advantages	Disadvantages
Medicine needs to be taken less regularly than tablets.	Injection may be painful.
Less likely to forget to have depot injection than tablets; therefore less likely to become ill or have a relapse.	Patient has less control over when to take their medicine; appointments dependent on availability of trained healthcare professionals.
Increased compliance/concordance due to decreased frequency of dosing.	Difficult to reverse the effects as medicine is administered in a slow-release formula.
Patient does not have any issues with storing medicines. However, as Davindra is homeless he could encounter problems trying to store his medicines safely, securely and in the right conditions.	Higher incidence of extrapyramidal reactions compared to oral administration.
Nobody (apart from his healthcare workers and whoever he chooses to tell) knows he is taking medicines.	Restlessness, dizziness, weight gain, blurred vision, stiffness in arms, legs, neck or mouth, tardive dyskinesia.

Activity 6.5 Healthcare inequalities and learning disabilities (page 157)

- People with learning disabilities have higher rates of certain medical conditions, such as diabetes, epilepsy, heart conditions and certain cancers (for example gastrointestinal cancers).
- People with learning disabilities often have communication difficulties.
- People with learning disabilities are more prone to poor health as a result of lower socioeconomic status and unemployment.
- There may be an inability to understand or assimilate fully health education advice such as that concerning cervical, prostate or breast cancer screening.
- There may be confusion among healthcare professionals regarding informed consent to treatment.
- Treatments associated with complex after-care or recovery regimens may not be offered to people with learning disabilities for fear they will be unable to comply fully.

Activity 6.6 Consent and learning disabilities (page 159)

- Ensure that Bill has the mental capacity to consent to be given his medicines.
- Ensure that he understands what you are telling him, by using language and terminology appropriate to his understanding. Use pictures, diagrams or symbols to aid his understanding if necessary.
- Ensure that he remembers what you are asking him to do, by asking questions to ascertain his understanding or asking him to explain to you what the treatment involves.
- Ensure that you have a clear response from Bill to signify he has agreed to the treatment (this can be by words, sign language, nodding of the head and so on).

Activity 6.7 Treatments for epilepsy (page 162)

- Sodium valproate: 1–2g in two daily divided doses (adults); 20–30mg/kg/day in two daily divided doses (children).
- Carbamazepine: 800mg–1.2g in two daily divided doses (adults); 5–10mg/kg/day in divided doses up to a maximum of 35mg/kg/day (children).
- A simple medicines regime may be easier for patients or their carers to understand and adhere to.
- There are fewer side effects and medicine interactions associated with single-dose medicines.

Activity 6.9 Asthma management poster (page 168)

The following are just some examples of the type of information that would be suitable:

- pictures of spacers and inhalers, and diagrams showing the correct techniques for using them;
- simple diagrams of the lungs and airways, and how asthma affects the airways;
- pictures or diagrams to show simple measures to take to reduce the risk of asthma attack, e.g regular exercise, washing cuddly toys, taking inhalers with children wherever they go.

Knowledge review

Now that you've worked through the chapter, how would you rate your knowledge of the following topics?

	Good	Adequate	Poor
1. Medical devices. 2. Management of diabetes mellitus. 3. Pain management in drug misusers. 4. Management of schizophrenia.			

	Good	Adequate	Poor
5. Obtaining informed consent in the learning disabilities patient. 6. Management of epilepsy. 7. Medicine dosages and concordance in children. 8. Asthma management.			

Where you're not confident in your knowledge of a topic, what will you do next?

Further reading

Blair, K (2011) *Medicines Management in Children's Nursing.* Exeter: Learning Matters.

A useful book that provides a good overview of a variety of medicines management issues in children's nursing.

Greenstein, B (2004). *Trounce's Clinical Pharmacology for Nurses.* 17th edition. Edinburgh: Churchill Livingstone.

This textbook provides useful overviews of clinical conditions such as schizophrenia, diabetes, asthma and epilepsy and their pharmacological management.

Jevon, P, Payne, E, Higgins, H and Endacott, R (2010) *Medicines Management: A guide for nurses.* Oxford: Wiley-Blackwell.

This is a practical textbook that offers plenty of information on various aspects of medicines management, particularly for adult and children's nurses.

Lawson, E and Hennefer, DL (2010) *Medicines Management in Adult Nursing.* Exeter: Learning Matters.

This book provides the reader with lots of useful information relevant to medicines management considerations in the adult patient.

Mutsatsa, S (2011) *Medicines Management in Mental Health Nursing.* Exeter: Learning Matters.

A practical book that offers plenty of information relating to a variety of medicines management issues in the patient with mental health problems.

Useful websites

http://asthma.org.uk

This website provides a wealth of information on asthma and its management.

www.diabetes.org.uk/Guide-to-diabetes/Introduction-to-diabetes

This website provides useful information on what diabetes is and its management.

www.epilepsysociety.org.uk

This website carries a variety of information on epilepsy and its management.

www.mencap.org

'The voice of learning disability', this website provides information particular to those with learning disabilities.

Chapter 7
Interprofessional roles in medicines management

continued . . .

By the second progression point:

2. Supports and assists others appropriately.

3. Values others' roles and responsibilities within the team and interacts appropriately.

4. Reflects on own practice and discusses issues with other members of the team to enhance learning.

Cluster: Medicines management

35. People can trust the newly registered graduate nurse to work as part of a team to offer holistic care and a range of treatment options of which medicines may form a part.

39. People can trust a newly registered graduate nurse to keep and maintain accurate records using information technology, where appropriate, within a multidisciplinary framework as a leader and as part of a team and in a variety of care settings including at home.

By the second progression point:

1. Demonstrates awareness of roles and responsibilities within the multidisciplinary team for medicines management, including how and in what ways information is shared within a variety of settings.

41. People can trust the newly registered graduate nurse to use and evaluate up-to-date information on medicines management and work within national and local policy guidelines.

By the second progression point:

1. Accesses commonly used evidence-based sources relating to the safe and effective management of medicine.

Chapter aims

By the end of this chapter, you should be able to:

- discuss the roles of the interprofessional team in medicines management;
- identify how interprofessional roles enhance the practices involved in medicines management.

Introduction

While Ian's poor progress is giving Bobbi and her staff cause for concern, there is a variety of experienced healthcare professionals available who can assist in resolving or managing his current problems. You will revisit this case later in the chapter to decide what input the various members of the interprofessional team have to ensure that Ian is well cared for.

Interprofessional working is essential in healthcare. You may be more familiar with the **interprofessional team** being referred to as the **multidisciplinary team (MDT)**. Both terms are used interchangeably and refer to the many different people who work within a healthcare environment, all with the aim of providing optimal care to patients. Using the term 'interprofessional' gives a stronger focus to the role that qualified and professionally regulated healthcare workers play. However, it is important to remember the vital role that non-qualified staff, such as healthcare assistants, domestics and porters also play in the delivery of high-quality patient care. Interprofessional working enables nurses and other professions allied to health to work together to ensure that patients receive the best care possible. This is vital in all areas of healthcare delivery.

Such an approach is seen as a key factor in improving medicines management (NIMHE National Workforce Programme, 2008). Over time it has become evident that there is a need for a collaborative approach to medicines management, whereby the skills and knowledge of different healthcare professionals can be brought together and utilised for best effect. Collaborative working aims to:

*   improve standards of patient care;
*   keep patients safe;
*   reduce the financial costs associated with the purchase and dispensing of medicines.

Creating a culture of teamwork and partnership in patient care will allow healthcare professionals to express any concerns they may have over the care of a patient, intervening when necessary, which should help to reduce any unintentional mistakes occurring in medicines management. It should also help to identify the very rare incidents where unscrupulous healthcare professionals do deliberate harm to patients. High-profile media cases such as that involving Harold Shipman, a GP who administered high doses of morphine to several elderly patients, which resulted in their premature deaths over a period of time, have highlighted the possible dangers of such healthcare professionals working in isolation. This chapter will explore the different interprofessional roles within healthcare and how people in these roles can work together to ensure that patients receive optimum care in medicines management. We shall explore how the traditional roles of the interprofessional team have evolved and advanced over time.

The interprofessional team

Historically, there has been a hierarchy of roles within healthcare and to some extent this still exists in our current healthcare system. Doctors were considered to have the most influence over patient care, their main role consisting of assessing, diagnosing and planning medical interventions. Their delivery of treatment tended to focus on more complex treatment regimens, for example ordering specialised investigations, performing surgical procedures and prescribing medicines – all roles associated with a higher level of responsibility and power. Nurses traditionally had a more subservient role of 'handmaiden' to the doctor and would deliver patient care according to the doctor's instructions. Procedures that were viewed as more simplistic and caring in nature were carried out by the nurse, for example administering injections, renewing surgical dressings and providing emotional comfort to patients. This led to a power imbalance between the two roles, which was further exacerbated by medicine being viewed as a profession and nursing a vocation. However, roles within the interprofessional team have evolved and continue to do so, with different professions realising that a collaborative approach to patient care is necessary to ensure that patients receive not only high-quality but also efficient and safe care. Mutual respect has grown over the years, coupled with changes in policy, education and legislation that have necessitated the need to work more closely together.

As a student nurse you are likely to come across situations where you see differences of opinion between members of the interprofessional team. This may be quite daunting for you, particularly if you are not sure who is 'right' and who is 'wrong'. The most important thing for you to remember is that the safety of your patients must always come first, regardless of the situation. Consider the dilemma facing the student nurse in the following activity.

You are on duty on the morning shift. You are caring for Hannah Bilboe, who is 22 and has learning disabilities. She has been admitted to your ward for 24 hours' observation with a minor head injury she sustained while suffering an epileptic fit. You and Hannah's mother are present in her cubicle with the doctor while she is being examined. Hannah's mother tells you and the doctor that her daughter has not had her anti-epileptic medicine this morning. She produces a box of tablets out of her handbag and asks the doctor if Hannah can be given her medicine.

The doctor replies 'Yes, of course. Give the box to the student nurse and she will give Hannah her usual dose.' The doctor turns to you and says 'I will be back later to write it up on the patient's drug chart.'

How would you respond to this request?

An outline answer is provided at the end of the chapter.

Working in partnership with each other is essential, with the patient being central in all decisions that are made. The sharing of information, knowledge and professional expertise should ensure that all patients receive optimum care in medicines management. Each professional has a responsibility to ensure that his or her actions do not lead or contribute to medicine errors. While it has already been highlighted in Chapter 1 that most errors occur at the administration stage, some may have been easily preventable at other stages of the medicines management process. One study estimates that 0.4 per cent of prescriptions contain errors that were identified and consequently averted by pharmacists. Administration errors occurred in approximately 5 per cent of all administered medicines on hospital wards (DH, 2004). In mental health nursing the importance of interprofessional working and patient involvement is recognised as a prerequisite to providing seamless care in medicines management (Healthcare Commission, 2007). Many examples from practice exist where patients have benefited from interprofessional working. In children's nursing, where many medicines are used outside their product licence, it is vital for professionals to work together to ensure safe doses are prescribed and administered.

Nurses

The roles and responsibilities of nurses in medicines management have already been discussed in Chapters 2, 5 and 6. Traditionally, their role has been confined to the administration stage. You may wish to refer back to Chapter 5 to re-examine the steps involved in the administration stage. However, with evolving and ever-expanding roles, nurses are increasingly being involved in prescribing medicines. Since nurses spend the majority of their time involved in direct patient care contact, more so than any other healthcare profession, it seems sensible that they should be involved with choosing the types of medicine their patients would benefit from. Studies have shown that nurses spend up to 40 per cent of their time administering medicines (Audit Commission, 2001).

As a student nurse you will have the opportunity to work with a variety of **nurse specialists**. These are registered nurses who have a wealth of experience and knowledge, and who have chosen to focus their experience and knowledge in a particular area of nursing. Often they are educated to Masters or PhD level, and have read and studied widely in their area of expertise. For example, you may be familiar with nurse specialists who deal in pain management or palliative care. They will work collaboratively with doctors and pharmacists, and be able to advise on the most effective ways to provide pain relief for patients or how best to manage the symptoms that a palliative care patient may be experiencing, such as nausea or vomiting. Increasingly, nurse specialists are taking on **independent prescribing** rights as well as supplementary prescribing and administering medicines under patient group directions (PGDs). These concepts are explored further in a free download on the website for this book at **www.learningmatters.co.uk/ nursing**.

As well as administering medicines to patients, the nurse is in an ideal position to notice any side effects or adverse reactions that the patient may suffer. This will enable the nurse to initiate prompt interventions to minimise any resultant harm to the patient.

It is worth remembering that with the ever-expanding role of the nurse come increasing levels of accountability and responsibility. In order to perform safe practice in medicines management and remain within legal, ethical and professional frameworks, registered nurses must ensure that they have the necessary competence and have been given the authority to administer or prescribe medicines. Here are some cases of nurses who have been referred to the NMC for failing to maintain professional requirements for medicines management.

Case study

A registered mental health nurse had a five-year **caution order** *placed on their registration due to numerous errors in recording and administering depot injections. On several occasions they chose to administer a depot injection, despite the prescription having been cancelled by the doctor.*

A registered adult nurse received a caution order of two years for several episodes of poor practice, including taking it upon themself to prescribe medicine to a patient. The NMC stated that the registrant was not legally entitled to write a prescription either by qualification or by subsequent training.

*(Source: **www.nmc-uk.org/Hearings/Hearings-and-outcomes**.)*

You may wish to go to the NMC website (see the case studies above), where you can read about more cases where nurses have been called to account for their actions or omissions in patient care. As a student nurse, in the event of your own competence or professionalism being called into question, you may be required to account for your actions by your university's fitness to practise panel or student conduct board. It is worth familiarising yourself with the various NMC codes and standards that registered nurses must adhere to; as a student nurse your university will be assessing and judging you against these standards.

Midwives

You may wonder why we are discussing the role of the midwife in medicines management. This is because, during your student nurse training, there will be occasions when you will work along-side midwives. Their role is to provide care to the expectant or new mother and their newborn babies. Often their role is very autonomous and, since pregnancy and childbirth are not illnesses but a normal part of life, many women choose to go through these processes with very little involvement from their doctors. Like nurses, midwives must adhere to the NMC's *Standards for Medicines Management* (NMC, 2007b). Midwives are also permitted to sell, supply and administer certain medicines that are exempt from restrictions under the Medicines Act 1968.

Doctors

The doctor's role in medicines management predominantly focuses on the prescribing of medicines. They need to have expert knowledge on the patient's condition in order to understand the most appropriate treatment options available to care for the patient. Doctors are expected to take a full patient history before prescribing any medicines. This history should include any previous or current medical conditions and any recently or currently used medicines. This should take account of any non-prescribed medicines such as herbal remedies, nutritional supplements, over-the-counter medicines (for example, cough syrups or paracetamol bought from a chemist) and any illegal substances.

Advances in the roles of the interprofessional team and legislation have had an impact on the roles and responsibilities of doctors. For example, the European Working Times Directive (Health and Safety Executive, 1998) limits the working week to 48 hours for junior doctors. This has resulted in a shift of some of the traditional roles and responsibilities of the doctor to the nurse. The Directive has expedited the expansion of the nurse's role in the prescribing of medicines.

It is worthwhile remembering that, just because the doctor has prescribed a medicine, registered nurses and student nurses must satisfy themselves that the prescription has been correctly written and it is appropriate for the patient. If you have any concerns about a prescription you must immediately bring it to the attention of the registered nurse and the prescriber.

Here are some true examples of the consequences of prescription errors.

Case study

A baby died after being prescribed and subsequently administered 12 times the usual dose of an anti-epileptic medicine.

(*Source:* Daily Mail Reporter, 2010.)

12 patients' deaths were attributed to a doctor for prescribing inappropriately wide dose ranges for opiates.

(*Source:* Greenhill, 2010.)

An elderly man died after being prescribed penicillin – a medicine he was allergic to.

(*Source:* Daily Mail Reporter, 2008.)

Like all healthcare professionals, doctors are also accountable for their actions and omissions, in law and professionally. Their professional regulator is the General Medical Council (GMC). As with the NMC, the GMC will hear cases of professional misconduct by doctors and make decisions based on whether any restrictions should be placed on a particular doctor's working practices. In very serious cases they may recommend that a doctor is struck off the register. If this happens, the doctor who is under investigation would not be able to practise medicine again in the UK. You may wish to read some of the cases that have been brought to the GMC, where a doctor's competence or professionalism has been called into question. You can do this by accessing the GMC's website given at the end of the chapter.

Pharmacists

The pharmacist's role is fundamental to every area of medicines management because he or she prepares and actually dispenses the medicines. Preparing and dispensing medicines is a key role and one that requires a great deal of knowledge, care and precision. The consequences of making mistakes in pharmacy can be catastrophic. Consider the following true cases.

Case study

A locum pharmacist dispensed propanolol instead of prednisolone to an elderly patient who subsequently died. The pharmacist received a suspended jail sentence.

(Source: Daily Mail Reporter, *2009.)*

A pharmacist dispensed sertraline instead of spironolactone to a patient with liver cancer. The patient died 22 days later. The pharmacist received a monetary fine as the medicine was not thought to have directly caused the patient's death.

(Source: Devine, *2008.)*

Often, only stories that result in a death are reported by the media. Patients who have been on the receiving end of medicine errors can become acutely ill and, in some cases, may have to live with the debilitating consequences of such errors for the rest of their lives. The Medicines Act 1968 classes dispensing errors as a criminal offence (HMSO, 1968). As we have seen from the case studies above, such errors can also have legal consequences for those who dispense medicines. The role of pharmacists is much more than simply dispensing medicines as per doctors' prescriptions. They are considered experts in medicines and their use, and are a valuable resource for any queries regarding medicines. Pharmacists work in several different areas: in hospitals, in the community or in primary care pharmacies. Some choose to work in areas outside the NHS, such as in industry (for example, pharmaceutical companies) or in education. Similarly to the nursing profession, pharmacists and pharmacy technicians must adhere to a code of ethics (RPSGB, 2007), which states that they must:

- make the care of patients their first concern;
- exercise professional judgement in the interests of patients and the public;

- show respect for others;
- encourage patients to participate in decisions about their care;
- develop their professional knowledge and competence;
- be honest and trustworthy;
- take responsibility for their working practices.

Pharmacists are a valuable resource to patients, nurses and other members of the interprofessional team. They are able to offer advice on the type of medicine, dosages, side effects and contra-indications. They must be knowledgeable in a variety of medical conditions in order to give advice on the most suitable and cost-effective medicine for a patient to be prescribed. Their contribution to quality control in reducing medicine errors is vital. Studies carried out by the Audit Commission (2001) highlighted that approximately 20–25 per cent of inpatient prescription charts needed amending by pharmacists due to errors in the basic rules of safe prescribing.

Activity 7.2   *Critical thinking*

Look closely at the patient medicine administration charts in Figures 7.1–7.3. What prescribing errors and poor practice in prescribing medicines would you expect a pharmacist to notice?

You may find it useful to have a BNF to hand to complete this activity.

An outline answer is provided at the end of the chapter.

A pharmacist can often be the first point of contact patients have with a healthcare professional when they are unwell. Consider the times you have been unwell and have gone to your local chemist or pharmacy for advice on how to best manage your complaint. They also offer advice on health promotion issues, for example smoking cessation. In order to qualify, pharmacists have to undergo a four-year pre-registration course at Masters level and undertake a one-year pre-registration period within a pharmacy.

Similar to nurses, pharmacists now have extended prescribing rights. In 2010, the General Pharmaceutical Council (GPhC) took over from the Royal Pharmaceutical Society of Great Britain (RPSGB) as the professional regulator for pharmacists, pharmacy technicians and pharmacy premises.

Dieticians

It may surprise you to learn that dieticians also have a role in medicines management. Their remit is usually limited to recommending food supplements for patients. While these may not be classified as medicines, they are often prescribed on the patient's medicine chart. Another area is that of weight management, not only through diet but also through weight loss management medicines. Dieticians are ideally placed in a medicines management role when patients' medicines regimes and dietary needs are fundamental to optimising their health. While it is not part of their role to be independent or supplementary prescribers, dieticians are able to issue certain medicines

Valley Hill NHS Foundation Trust

SURNAME Abdi	FORENAME Rahman	DATE OF BIRTH 12/07/2003 7 years and 3 months	PATIENT IDENTIFICATION NUMBER 120967	ALLERGIES None known
HEIGHT 1.2m	WEIGHT 21kg	CONSULTANT Saiko	SPECIAL DIETARY REQUIREMENTS None	

ONCE ONLY DRUGS/VARIABLE DOSE PRESCRIPTIONS

Date	Drug	Dose	Route	Prescriber's signature	Administered by	Date and time	Pharmacy

REGULAR PRESCRIPTIONS

	Time														Date			

Drug Amoxicillin — 06.00

Route	Dose	Start Date	End Date	Time 12.00
0	350mg	10/10/10	15/10/10	

Prescriber's Signature *R Halls* — Pharmacy — 18.00 / 24.00

Drug Beta-Cardone® — 06.00

Route	Dose	Start Date	End Date
0	40mg	10/10/10	15/10/10

Prescriber's Signature *R Halls* — Pharmacy — 18.00

Drug Bisacodyl — 08.00

Route	Dose	Start Date	End Date
0	5	10/10/10	15/10/10

Prescriber's Signature *R Halls* — Pharmacy — 20.00

Figure 7.1: Patient medicine administration charts showing errors

Valley Hill NHS Foundation Trust

SURNAME Rosario	FORENAME Dexter	DATE OF BIRTH 29/10/29	PATIENT IDENTIFICATION NUMBER 397856	ALLERGIES Penicillin
HEIGHT 1.7m	WEIGHT 73kg	CONSULTANT Decouto	SPECIAL DIETARY REQUIREMENTS None	

ONCE ONLY DRUGS/VARIABLE DOSE PRESCRIPTIONS

Date	Drug	Dose	Route	Prescriber's signature	Administered by	Date and time	Pharmacy

REGULAR PRESCRIPTIONS

				Time	Date										
Drug Paracetamol				06.00											
				12.00											
Route O	Dose 1g	Start Date 10/10/10	End Date 15/10/10	14.00											
				18.00											
Prescriber's Signature B Morris		Pharmacy		20.00											
				24.00											
Drug Zopiclone				06.00											
Route O	Dose 7.5mg	Start Date 10/10/10	End Date 15/10/10												
Prescriber's Signature B Morris		Pharmacy													
Drug Digoxin				08.00											
Route O	Dose .625mg	Start Date 10/10/10	End Date 15/10/10												
Prescriber's Signature B Morris		Pharmacy													

Figure 7.2: Patient medicine administration charts showing errors

Valley Hill NHS Foundation Trust

SURNAME Sacker	FORENAME Riordan	DATE OF BIRTH 19/11/55	PATIENT IDENTIFICATION NUMBER 290900	ALLERGIES Cyclizine
HEIGHT 1.65m	WEIGHT 81kg	CONSULTANT Bosworth	SPECIAL DIETARY REQUIREMENTS None	

ONCE ONLY DRUGS/VARIABLE DOSE PRESCRIPTIONS

Date	Drug	Dose	Route	Prescriber's signature	Administered by	Date and time	Pharmacy
10/10/10	Heparin	5000 units	S.C	Sandrea Daval	J Taylor	10/10/10 at 05.55	

REGULAR PRESCRIPTIONS

				Time	Date										
Drug Gliclazide															
Route O	Dose 80mg	Start Date 10/10/10	End Date 15/10/10	15.00											
Prescriber's Signature Sandrea Daval		Pharmacy													
Drug Co-codamol				06.00											
Route O	Dose 2 tabs	Start Date 10/10/10	End Date 15/10/10	12.00 18.00											
Prescriber's Signature Sandrea Daval		Pharmacy		24.00											
Drug Paracetamol				06.00											
Route O	Dose 1g	Start Date 10/10/10	End Date 15/10/10	12.00											
Prescriber's Signature Sandrea Daval		Pharmacy		18.00 20.00											

Figure 7.3: Patient medicine administration charts showing errors

under PGDs. An important role of the dietician is to be aware of possible interactions between the medicines patients are receiving and their diets. These are commonly called **food–drug interactions**. We have seen from Chapter 3 that some medicines should not be given together as they may interact with each other; the same can apply to foods. Dieticians should therefore know what medicines a patient is receiving, alert the patient and relevant healthcare professionals of any possible food–drug interactions and make recommendations such as not administering certain medicines with food. Please note that their responsibility for this will be limited to those patients who have been referred to them for dietary management. Their professional regulator is the Health Professions Council (HPC). Like other registered healthcare professionals, any allegations made against dieticians are handled by the fitness to practise department of their regulatory body.

Non-qualified healthcare workers

It is important not to forget the vital role that non-qualified healthcare workers play in medicines management. Healthcare assistants (HCAs) are often delegated the responsibility of administering medicines to patients who live in residential homes or require assistance with their medicines from a community HCA/Support Worker. The NMC (2007b, p52) offers clear guidance regarding responsibility and accountability issues. They state the following:

> In delegating the administration of medicinal products to unregistered practitioners, it is the registrant who must apply the principles of administration of medicinal products . . . They may then delegate an unregistered practitioner to assist the patient in the ingestion or application of the medicinal product.

In essence this means that HCAs are responsible for their actions and any resultant consequences of them when giving patients in their care their medicines, but the ultimate accountability for their actions lies with the registered nurse. It is therefore essential for HCAs to receive training in medicines administration.

Other non-qualified members of the healthcare team also play a role. For example, in a hospital setting porters will often transport medicines between the pharmacy and the ward or department. Domestics and housekeepers should notify nursing staff of any medicines found on the floor during their cleaning duties.

Activity 7.3 — *Team working*

Now go back to the case study at the beginning of the chapter. What action or input do you think the various members of the interprofessional team might have in Ian's care?

An outline answer is provided at the end of the chapter.

Now that we have explored the roles and responsibilities of the interprofessional team in medicines management, you should be aware of the differences and similarities that exist within the different healthcare professions. The prescribing and administration rights of the interprofessional team are explored further in a free download on the website for this book at **www.learning matters.co.uk/nursing**.

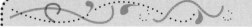

Chapter summary

You have learnt from this chapter that interprofessional working is vital as a means of sharing important advice and information that will impact on the medicines that are prescribed for your patients. We have explored how healthcare professionals can work alongside each other to enhance the patient experience without compromising their own professional identity. A mutual respect and understanding for each other's roles will do much to ensure that a patient-centred approach to medicines management is taken. Examples of areas of, and the consequences of, poor medicines management have been highlighted, for both the healthcare professional and the patient. A collaborative approach to this important aspect of patient care will not only advance your knowledge but also increase patient safety and improve patient care.

Activities: brief outline answers

Activity 7.1 Student nurse asked to administer medicine (page 176)

You should ask the doctor if you could speak to him/her away from the patient's cubicle. You should politely excuse yourself from Hannah and her mother, explaining that you will be back with them very shortly. In a quiet area you should explain to the doctor that, as a student nurse, you are unable to administer any medicines to a patient without the direct supervision of a registered nurse. You should explain to the doctor that, in order for Hannah to be administered her medicine straightaway, the doctor should prescribe it on the patient's prescription chart now. Once this is done you should inform the doctor that you will take the chart to a staff nurse who will then be able to supervise you in dispensing and administering the medicine to Hannah.

Activity 7.2 Errors in patient medicine adminstration charts (page 180)

The pharmacist in reviewing the charts should have noticed the following prescribing errors/poorly written prescriptions and contacted the prescriber to amend or rewrite the prescriptions:

Rahman Abdi's chart (7.1) (page 181)

- The dose and frequency of amoxicillin does not follow the recommended guidelines stated in the BNF. The usual dose for children up to the age of ten years is 125mg every eight hours, doubled in severe infections. Therefore, the incorrect dose has been prescribed and the frequency should be three times a day and not four times a day as indicated on the prescription.
- Beta-Cardone is a trade or brand name of a medicine called sotalol hydrochloride. It is considered best practice to prescribe a medicine using its generic name.
- The unit of weight for bisacodyl has not been prescribed. It should read 5mg.

Dexter Rosario's chart (7.2) (page 182)

- The frequency of doses for paracetamol is incorrect. The maximum frequency is every 4–6 hours with a maximum dose of 4g in 24 hours.
- The time prescribed for zopiclone to be administered is incorrect. It should be prescribed for administration at night time.
- The dose of digoxin is poorly prescribed. It should be prescribed in micrograms rather than grams to reduce the risk of overdose. It should be prescribed as 62.5mcg and not .0625mg. The decimal point is not obvious.

Riordan Sacker's chart (7.3) (page 183)

- Gliclazide should be taken with breakfast.
- Co-codamol is manufactured in several different dose strengths. The pharmacist should ask the doctor to prescribe the dose strength he or she wishes the patient to be given (for example, 8/500, 15/500 or 30/500).
- Paracetamol has been prescribed, but the patient cannot take this and co-codamol since each co-codamol tablet contains 500mg of paracetamol. For both prescriptions the maximum dose of paracetamol has been prescribed. The pharmacist should ask the doctor to discontinue one of the prescriptions.

Activity 7.3 Interprofessional input into patient care (page 184)

The senior staff nurse should ensure that appropriate referrals are made to the interprofessional team, communicate Ian's progress to those involved in his care, inform staff looking after Ian of changes in his care plan and so forth, and inform his next of kin as to how he is progressing. Covert administration of his medicines may be discussed.

The pharmacist will review Ian's medicine regimen. It may be appropriate to offer an alternative preparation for his medicine. For example, he may be spitting out his medicine because he doesn't like taking tablets.

The orthopaedic consultant may decide to order additional investigations (for example, an X-ray to check that the dynamic hip screw is fixed appropriately) or perform a thorough physical examination of Ian.

The dietician, in conjunction with nursing staff will carry out a full nutritional assessment of Ian. He may suggest that Ian is referred to the speech and language therapist for swallowing tests, as he is not taking his tablets and is eating very little. He may decide to offer food supplements to Ian and recommend that nursing staff maintain an accurate food intake chart for him.

The physiotherapist, in conjunction with nursing staff, will carry out a mobility assessment on Ian. She may help Ian with passive or active limb exercises while he is unable to get out of bed, ensuring that he receives analgesia prior to these exercises. She may also perform chest physio to help him expectorate any chest secretions.

The learning disabilities nurse and social worker will communicate with Ian in an appropriate manner that will allow him the opportunity to understand and give informed consent to any care or treatment. They will also advise the nursing staff on any particular communication techniques that would enhance therapeutic interactions between themselves and Ian. They will also make recommendations for any discharge planning.

The occupational therapist will assess Ian's ability to perform activities of daily living, once he is more mobile, to ensure that he has the opportunity to return to as independent a living style as he can.

Knowledge review

Now that you've worked through the chapter, how would you rate your knowledge of the following topics?

	Good	Adequate	Poor
1. Roles and responsibilities of the interprofessional team in medicines management.			

Where you're not confident in your knowledge of a topic, what will you do next?

Further reading

Department of Health (DH) (2006) *Improving Patients' Access to Medicines: A guide to implementing nurse and pharmacist independent prescribing within the NHS in England*. London: Department of Health.

This is a useful document that discusses non-medical prescribing.

Department of Health (DH) (2006) *Medicines Matters: A guide to mechanisms for the prescribing, supply and administration of medicines*. London: Department of Health.

This document deals with prescribing, supplying and administration issues relating to medicines.

Useful websites

www.gmc-uk.org/concerns/hearings_and_decisions/fitness_to_practise_decisions.asp

This website will allow you to learn about doctors who have been referred to the GMC for competence or professionalism concerns.

www.nhsbsa.nhs.uk/PrescriptionServices/Documents/PrescriptionServices/Current_and_Out_of_Date_Rx_Form_Published_0709.pdf

This website will enable you to see the current prescription forms that are used in practice.

www.nmc-uk.org/Hearings/Hearings-and-outcomes

You can access this website to read about nurses who have been referred to the NMC when their competence or professionalism has been called into question.

www.learningmatters.co.uk/nursing

Visit the website for this book by clicking on 'Full list of nursing and midwifery titles'. Then click on Introduction to Medicines Management in Nursing. This webpage contains a free download exploring Patient Group Directions and Non-Medical Prescribing. You can also access a glossary for the book from this webpage.

References

Anderson, S (ed.) (2005) *Making Medicines: A brief history of pharmacy and pharmaceuticals.* London: Pharmaceutical Press.

Associated Press (2009) Experts: placebo power behind many natural cures. *Associated Press*, 10 November. Available online at www.foxnews.com/story/0,2933,573846,00.html (accessed 25 October 2010).

Asthma UK (2010) *What is Asthma?* Available online at www.asthma.org.uk/all_about_asthma/asthma_basics/index.html (accessed 30 September 2010).

Audit Commission (2001) *A Spoonful of Sugar.* London: Audit commission. Available online at www.audit commission.gov.uk/nationalstudies/health/other/pages/aspoonfulofsugar.aspx (accessed 22 August 2010).

Bernal, J (2003) *Epilepsy: Learning about intellectual disabilities and health.* Available online at www.intellectual disability.info/physical-health/epilepsy (accessed 25 July 2010).

British National Formulary (BNF) (2010) *BNF 59.* London: BMJ Group/Pharmaceutical Press. Available online at www.bnf.org/bnf/ (accessed 30 August 2010).

British National Formulary for Children (BNFC) (2009) London: BMJ Group/Pharmaceutical Press.

Carr, ECJ, Thomas, VJ and Wilson-Barnett, J (2005) Patient experiences of anxiety, depression and acute pain after surgery. *International Journal of Nursing Studies*, 42: 521–30.

Chao, MT and Wade, CM (2008) Socioeconomic factors and women's use of complementary and alternative medicine in four racial/ethnic groups. *Ethnicity & Disease*, 18: 65–71.

Cramer, H, Shaw, A, Wye, L and Weiss, M (2010) Over-the-counter advice about seeking complementary and alternative medicines (CAMs) in community pharmacies and health shops: an ethnographic study. *Health and Social Care in the Community*, 18(1): 41–50.

Daily Mail Reporter (2008) Patient 'killed by GP who ignored penicillin allergy warning'. Mail Online. Available online at www.dailymail.co.uk/news/article-1086689/patient-killed-GP-ignored-penicillin-allergy-warning-html (accessed 8 January 2011).

Daily Mail Reporter (2009) Grandmother died after Tesco chemist accidentally gave her the wrong pills. Mail Online. Available online at www.dailymail.co.uk/news/article-1166822/pensioner-died-Tesco-chemist-accidentally-gave-wrong-pills-html (accessed 8 January 2011).

Daily Mail Reporter (2010) Baby dies after blundering doctors gave him twelve times the normal dose of epilepsy drugs. Mail Online. Available online at www.dailymail.co.uk/news/article-1289437/Baby-died-doctors-gave-12-times-normal-dose-epilespy-drugs-html (accessed 8 January 2011).

Department of Health (DH) (1989) *Report of the Advisory Group on Nurse Prescribing (Crown report).* London: HMSO.

Department of Health (DH) (1997a) Children Act 1989; Guidance and regulations. London: HMSO

Department of Health (DH) (1997b) *Prescription Fraud Efficiency Scrutiny Report.* London: HMSO.

Department of Health (DH) (2000) *An Organisation with a Memory.* London: The Stationery Office.

Department of Health (DH) (2001a) *Patients to Get Quicker Access to Medicines* (press release). London: Department of Health.

Department of Health (DH) (2001b) *Medicines and Older People: Implementing medicines related aspects of the NSF for older people.* Available online at www.dh.gov.uk/prod_consum_dh/groups/dh_digitalassets/@dh/@en/documents/digitalasset/dh_4067247.pdf (accessed 30 September 2010).

Department of Health (DH) (2001c) *Valuing People: A new strategy for learning disability for the 21st century* (white paper). London: The Stationery Office.

Department of Health (DH) (2004) *Building a Safer NHS for Patients: Improving medication safety.* Available online at www.dh.gov.uk/dr_consum_dh/groups/dh_digitalassets/@dh/@en/documents/digitalasset/dh_408 4961.pdf (accessed 22 August 2010).

Department of Health (DH) (2005) *Supplementary Prescribing by Nurses, Pharmacists, Chiropodists/Podiatrists, Physiotherapists and Radiographers within the NHS in England: A guide for implementation.* London: The Stationery Office.

Department of Health (DH) (2006) *Safer Management of Controlled Drugs: Guidance on standard operating procedures for controlled drugs.* London: Department of Health.

Department of Health (DH) (2007a) *Safer Management of Controlled Drugs: Early action.* Available online at www.dh.gov.uk/en/Healthcare/Medicinespharmacyandindustry/Prescriptions/DH_4123320 (accessed 4 November 2010).

Department of Health (DH) (2007b) *Reference Guide to Consent for Examination or Treatment.* Available online at www.dh.gov.uk/prod_consum_dh/groups/dh_digitalassets/documents/digitalasset/dh_103653.pdf (accessed 13 September 2010).

Department of Health (DH) (2008) *Healthcare for All: Report of the independent inquiry into access to healthcare for people with learning disabilities.* Available online at www.dh.gov.uk/prod_consum_dh/groups/dh_digital assets/@dh/@en/documents/digitalasset/dh_106126.pdf (accessed 3 December 2010).

Department of Health (DH) (2009) *Records Management: NHS Code of Practice: Part 2*, 2nd edition. Available online at www.dh.gov.uk/prod_consum_dh/groups/dh_digitalassets/documents/digitalasset/dh_0930 24.pdf (accessed 7 September 2010).

Devine, D. (2008) Fined pharmacists gave wrong drug to patient who died. Wales news. Available online at www.walesonline.co.uk/news/wales-news/2008/09/06/fined-pharmacists-gave-wrong-drug-to-patient-who-died-91466-21685354/ (accessed 8 January 2011).

Diabetes UK (2010a) *What is Type 1 Diabetes?* Available online at www.diabetes.org.uk/Guide-to-diabetes/ Introduction-to-diabetes/What_is_diabetes/What-is-Type-1-diabetes/ (accessed 30 September 2010).

Diabetes UK (2010b) *What is Type 2 Diabetes?* Available online at www.diabetes.org.uk/Guide-to-diabetes/Introduction-to-diabetes/What_is_diabetes/What-is-Type-2-diabetes/ (accessed 30 September 2010).

Dougherty, L and Lister, S (2008) Drug administration: delivery (infusion devices), in *The Royal Marsden Hospital Manual of Clinical Nursing Procedures: Student edition*, 7th edition. Oxford: Wiley-Blackwell.

Eccleston, C, Malleson, PN, Clinch, J, Connell, H and Sourbut, C (2003) Chronic pain in adolescents: evaluation of a programme of interdisciplinary cognitive behaviour therapy. *Archives of Diseases in Childhood*, 88: 881–5.

Edirne, T, Gunher Arica, S, Gucuk, S, Yildizhan, R, Kolusari, A, Adali, E and Can, M (2010) Use of complementary and alternative medicines by a sample of Turkish women for infertility enhancement: a descriptive study. *BMC Complementary and Alternative Medicine*, 10: 11.

Edwards, RR, Doleys, DM, Fillingim, RB and Lowery, B (2001) Ethnic differences in pain tolerance: clinical implications in a chronic pain population. *Psychosomatic Medicine*, 63: 316–23.

Ernst, E, Resch, KL, Mills, S, Hill, R, Mitchell, A, Willoughby, M and White, A (1995) Complementary medicine – a definition. *British Journal of General Practice*, 45: 506.

Galbraith, A, Bullock, S, Manias, E, Hunt, B and Richards, A (2007) *Fundamentals of Pharmacology: An applied approach for nursing and health*, 2nd edition. London: Prentice Hall.

Greenhill, S (2010) Fury as doctor of death is told: carry on practising. Mail Online. Available online at www.dailymail.co.uk/news/article-1247000/Dr-Jane-Barton-escapes-struck-prescribing-potentially-hazardous-levels-drugs-html (accessed 8 January 2011).

Griffith, R and Tengnah, C (2010) *Law and Professional Issues in Nursing*, 2nd edition. Exeter: Learning Matters.

Health and Safety Executive (HSE) (1998) *The Working Time Regulations 1998*. Available online at www.hse.gov.uk/contact/faqs/workingtimedirective.htm (accessed 30 August 2010).

Healthcare Commission (2007) Talking about medicines: the management of medicines in trusts providing mental health services. London. Commission for healthcare audit and inspection.

HMSO (1968) *Medicines Act 1968*. London: HMSO. Available online at www.statutelaw.gov.uk/AZIndex.aspx (accessed 10 September 2010).

HMSO (1971) *Misuse of Drugs Act 1971*. London: HMSO. Available online at www.statutelaw.gov.uk/AZ Index.aspx (accessed 13 September 2010).

HMSO (1973/2001) *Misuse of Drugs Regulations 1973/2001*. London: HMSO. Available online at www.legislation.gov.uk/uksi/2001/3998/contents/made (accessed 7 November 2010).

HMSO (1973/2007) *Misuse of Drugs (Safe Custody) Regulations 1973/2007*. Available online at www.statutelaw.gov.uk (accessed 10 November 2010).

HMSO (1983) *Mental Health Act 1983*. Available online at www.cqc.org.uk/_db/_documents/Mental_Health_Act_1983_201005272747.pdf (accessed 30 September 2010).

HMSO (1992) *Medicinal Products: Prescription by Nurse etc. Act 1992*. London: HMSO.

HMSO (1995) *Disability Discrimination Act 1995*. Available online at: www.legislation.gov.uk/ukpga/1995/50/contents (accessed 13 December 2010).

HMSO (1998) *Data Protection Act 1998*. Available online at www.legislation.gov.uk/ukpga/1998/29/contents (accessed 9 September 2010).

HMSO (2005) *Mental Capacity Act 2005*. Available online at www.legislation.gov.uk/ukpga/2005/9/contents (accessed 13 December 2010).

HMSO (2006) *Controlled Drugs (Supervision of Management and Use) Regulations 2006*. Available online at www.legislation.gov.uk/uksi/2006/3148/contents/made (accessed 7 November 2010).

HMSO (2007) *Mental Health Act 2007*. Available online at www.legislation.gov.uk/ukpga/2007/12 (accessed 13 December 2010).

Hoare, J and Flatley, J (2008) *Drug Misuse Declared: Findings from the 2007/8 British Crime Survey, England and Wales*. London: Home Office Statistics.

Hollins, S, Attard, MT, von Fraunhofer, N and Sedgwick, O (1998) Mortality in people with learning disabilities: risks, causes and death certification findings in London. *Developmental Medicine and Child Neurology*, 40: 50–6.

House of Lords Select Committee on Science and Technology (2000) *Complementary and Alternative Medicine*. HL Paper 123, November. London: The Stationery Office.

Kronenburg, F, Cushman, LF, Wade, CM, Kalmuss, D and Chao, MT (2006) Race/ethnicity and women's use of complementary and alternative medicine in the United States: results of a national survey. *American Journal of Public Health*, 96(7): 1236–42.

Lee, PT (2010) A team approach to identify and manage risk in infusion therapy. *British Journal of Nursing*, 19(5): S12–18.

Lorenc, A, Ilan-Clarke, Y, Robinson, N and Blair, M (2009) How parents choose to use CAM: a systematic review of theoretical models. *BMC Complementary and Alternative Medicine*, 9: 9.

Medical Devices Agency (2003) *Infusion Systems*. Available online at www.mhra.gov.uk (accessed 30 July 2010).

Medicines and Healthcare products Regulatory Agency (MHRA). *Who We Are*. Accessed online at: www.mhra.gov.uk/Aboutus/Whoweare/index.htm (accessed 10 December 2010).

Melzack, R and Wall, P (1965) Pain mechanism: a new theory. *Science*, 150: 971–9.

Mencap (2004) *Treat Me Right: Better health care for people with a learning disability*. Available online at www.mencap.org.uk/document.asp?id=316 (accessed 13 September 2010).

Mencap (2007) *Death by Indifference: Following up the Treat Me Right report*. Available online at www.mencap.org.uk/page.asp?id=9604 (accessed 13 September 2010).

Moore, RA, Tramer, MR and McQuay, HJ (1997) Transcutaneous electrical nerve stimulation does not relieve labour pain: updated systematic review. *Contemporary Reviews in Obstetrics and Gynecology*, 195–205.

Mosteller, RD (1987) Simplified calculation of body surface area. *New England Journal of Medicine*, 317: 1098.

National Health Service (NHS) (2010a) *NHS Choices: Epilepsy*. Available online at www.nhs.uk/Conditions/Epilepsy/Pages/Causes.aspx (accessed 10 September 2010).

National Health Service (NHS) (2010b) *NHS Choices: Schizophrenia*: Available online at www.nhs.uk/Conditions/Schizophrenia/Pages/Symptoms.aspx (accessed 13 September 2010).

National Institute for Health and Clinical Excellence (NICE) (2000). *Guidance on the Use of Inhaler Systems (Devices) in Children under the Age of 5 years with Chronic Asthma*. Available online at www.nice.org.uk/nicemedia/live/11400/32073/32073.pdf (accessed 7 November 2010).

National Institute for Health and Clinical Excellence (NICE) (2003) *Infection Control Prevention of Healthcare-associated Infection in Primary and Community Care*. London: NICE.

National Institute for Health and Clinical Excellence (NICE) (2008) *Drug Misuse: Psychosocial interventions*. National Clinical Practice Guidelines Number 51. London: NICE. Available online at www.nice.org.uk/nicemedia/live/11812/35975/35975.pdf (accessed 6 September 2010).

National Patient Safety Agency (NPSA) (2009) *Safety in Doses: Improving the use of medicines in the NHS*. London: National Patient Safety Agency.

National Prescribing Centre (2009) *Patient Group Directions: A practical guide and framework of competencies for all professionals using patient group directions*. Available online at www.npc.co.uk/prescribers/resources/patient_group_directions.pdf (accessed 30 August 2010).

NIMHE National Workforce Programme (2008) *Medicines Management: Everybody's business*. London: Department of Health.

NSPCC (1985) *What is Gillick Competency? What are the Fraser Guidelines?* Available online at www.nspcc.org.uk/inform/research/questions/gillick_wda61289.html (accessed 4 November 2010).

Nurse Prescribers' Formulary (NPF) (2009) *Nurse Prescribers' Formulary for Community Practitioners 2009–2011*. London: BMJ Group/Pharmaceutical Press. Available online at http://bnf.org/bnf/extra/current/popup/NPF2009-2011.pdf (accessed 8 August 2010).

Nursing and Midwifery Council (NMC) (2006) *Standards of Proficiency for Nurse and Midwife Prescribers*. London: NMC.

Nursing and Midwifery Council (NMC) (2007a) *Covert Administration of Medicines: Disguising medicine in food and drink*. Available online at www.nmc-uk.org/Nurses-and-midwives/Advice-by-topic/A/Advice/Covert-administration-of-medicines/ (accessed 13 September 2010).

Nursing and Midwifery Council (NMC) (2007b) *Standards for Medicines Management*. London: NMC.

Nursing and Midwifery Council (NMC) (2008) *The Code: Standards of conduct, performance and ethics for nurses and midwives*. London: NMC.

Nursing and Midwifery Council (NMC) (2009) *Record Keeping: Guidance for nurses and midwives*. London: NMC.

Nursing and Midwifery Council (NMC) (2010a) *Standards for Pre-registration Nursing Education*. London: NMC.

Nursing and Midwifery Council (NMC) (2010b) *Guidance on Professional Conduct for Nursing and Midwifery Students*. Available online at www.nmc-uk.org/Documents/Guidance/Guidance-on-professional-conduct-for-nursing-and-midwifery-students-September-2010.PDF (accessed 7 November 2010).

Resuscitation Council (UK) (2008) *Emergency Treatment of Anaphylactic Reactions*. London: Resuscitation Council. Available online at www.resus.org.uk/pages/reaction.pdf (accessed 7 November 2010).

Reveley, S (1998) The role of the triage nurse practitioner in general medical practice: an analysis of the role. *Journal of Advanced Nursing*, 28(3): 584–91.

Royal College of Nursing (RCN) (2006) *Patient Group Directions: Guidance and information for nurses*. London: RCN. Available online at www.rcn.org.uk/_data/assets/pdf_file/0008/78506/001370.pdf (accessed 7 August 2010).

Royal Pharmaceutical Society of Great Britain (RPSGB) (2007) *Code of Ethics for Pharmacists and Pharmacy Technicians*. London: Royal Pharmaceutical Society of Great Britain.

Seamark, M (2008) 'Wrong' woman given abortion after nurse mixed up patients. Available online at www.dailymail.co.uk/news/article-1036284 (accessed 7 January 2010).

Searson, B (2008) Meeting the challenges of epilepsy. *Learning Disability Practice*, 11(9): 29–35.

Shipman Enquiry Reports (2002–5) *Fourth Report – The Regulation of Controlled Drugs in the Community*, published 15 July 2004, Command Paper Cm 6249. London: The Stationery Office. Available online at www.the-shipman-inquiry.org.uk/reports.asp (accessed 7 November 2010).

Stokes, T, Shaw, EJ, Juarez-Garcia, A, Camosso-Stefinovic, J and Baker, R (2004) *Clinical Guidelines and Evidence Review for the Epilepsies: Diagnosis and management in adults and children in primary and secondary care*. London: Royal College of Physicians.

Thomas, V (2007) The management of pain, in Walsh, M and Crumbie, A (eds) *Watson's Clinical Nursing and Related Sciences*. Edinburgh: Bailliere Tindall.

Torrence, C (1989) Intramuscular injection, part 1 and 2. *Surgical Nurses*, 2(5): 6–10, 2(6): 24–7.

World Health Organization (WHO) (2010) *Lexicon of Alcohol and Drug Terms*. Available online at www.who.int/substance_abuse/terminology/who_lexicon/en/print.html (accessed 13 September 2010).

Index